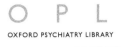

OXFORD PSYCHIATRY LIBRARY

CW00816192

Treatment Response and Resistance in Schizophrenia

O P L

OXFORD PSYCHIATRY LIBRARY

Treatment Response and Resistance in Schizophrenia

Edited by

Oliver Howes

Professor of Molecular Psychiatry
King's College London, London, UK
Institute of Medical Sciences, Imperial College London
Maudsley Hospital, London, UK

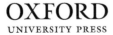

OXFORD
UNIVERSITY PRESS

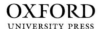

OXFORD
UNIVERSITY PRESS

Great Clarendon Street, Oxford, OX2 6DP,
United Kingdom

Oxford University Press is a department of the University of Oxford.
It furthers the University's objective of excellence in research, scholarship,
and education by publishing worldwide. Oxford is a registered trade mark of
Oxford University Press in the UK and in certain other countries

First Edition published in 2018

Impression: 2

Published in the United States of America by Oxford University Press
198 Madison Avenue, New York, NY 10016, United States of America

British Library Cataloguing in Publication Data
Data available

Library of Congress Control Number: 2018949666

ISBN 978–0–19–882876–1

Printed by
CPI Group (UK) Ltd, Croydon CR0 4YY

Oxford University Press makes no representation, express or implied, that the
drug dosages in this book are correct. Readers must therefore always check
the product information and clinical procedures with the most up-to-date
published product information and data sheets provided by the manufacturers
and the most recent codes of conduct and safety regulations. The authors and
the publishers do not accept responsibility or legal liability for any errors in the
text or for the misuse or misapplication of material in this work. Except where
otherwise stated, drug dosages and recommendations are for the non-pregnant
adult who is not breast-feeding

Links to third party websites are provided by Oxford in good faith and
for information only. Oxford disclaims any responsibility for the materials
contained in any third party website referenced in this work.

Contents

Abbreviations

ACE	angiotensin-converting enzyme
ANC	absolute neutrophil count
APD	antipsychotic drug
AVATAR	audiovisual-assisted therapy aid for refractory auditory hallucinations
BDNF	brain-derived neurotrophic factor
BEN	benign ethnic neutropenia
BMI	body mass index
BPRS	Brief Psychiatric Rating Scale
CATIE	Clinical Antipsychotic Trials of Intervention Effectiveness
CBC	complete blood count
CBD	cannabidiol
CBTp	cognitive behaviour therapy for psychosis
CES	clozapine-eligible schizophrenia
CGI-S	Clinical Global Impression–Severity
CGI-SCH	Clinical Global Impression–Schizophrenia
CI	confidence interval
CIAS	cognitive impairment associated with schizophrenia
CNS	central nervous system
CR	cognitive remediation
CRS	clozapine-resistant schizophrenia
CT	computed tomography
D2R	dopamine D2 receptor
DALY	disability-adjusted life year
DHEA	dehydroepiandrosterone
dTDP	torsade de pointes
ECG	electrocardiogram
ECT	electroconvulsive therapy
EE	expressed emotion
EOI	emotional overinvolvement
EPS	extrapyramidal side effect
FDA	Food and Drug Administration
FES	first episode of schizophrenia
FGA	first-generation antipsychotics
GABA	gamma-aminobutyric acid
GAF	global assessment of function

IL	interleukin
INF	interferon
KAT	kynurenine aminotransferase
KYNA	kynurenic acid
LSD	lysergic acid diethylamide
MRI	magnetic resonance imaging
MRS	magnetic resonance spectroscopy
NAC	N-acetylcysteine
nAChRs	nicotinic acetylcholine receptors
NCR	not criminally responsible
NICE	National Institute for Health and Care Excellence
NMDA	N-methyl-D-aspartate
NSAID	non-steroidal anti-inflammatory drug
PANSS	Positive And Negative Syndrome Scale
PCP	phencyclidine
PET	positron emission tomography
pHVA	plasma homovanillic acid
RCT	randomized controlled trial
RDoC	Research Domain Criteria
REMS	Risk Evaluation and Mitigation Strategy
rTMS	repetitive transcranial magnetic stimulation
SANS	Scale for the Assessment of Negative Symptoms
SAPS	Scale for the Assessment of Positive Symptoms
SGA	second-generation antipsychotic
SMD	standardized mean difference
SNRI	serotonin–norepinephrine reuptake inhibitor
SOFAS	Social and Occupational Functioning Scale
SPECT	single photon emission computed tomography
SSRI	selective serotonin reuptake inhibitor
SUCRA	surface under the cumulative ranking curve
tDCS	transcranial direct current stimulation
TD	tardive dyskinesia
TGF	transforming growth factor
TRRIP	Treatment Response and Resistance in Psychosis
TRS	treatment-resistant schizophrenia
URS	ultra-resistant schizophrenia
VHA	Veterans Health Administration

Contributors

Ofer Agid

Schizophrenia Program
Centre for Addiction and Mental
Health (CAMH)
and Department of Psychiatry,
Faculty of Medicine,
University of Toronto,
Toronto, Canada

Thomas R. E. Barnes

Imperial College London, London, UK

Majella Byrne

Psychological Interventions Clinic for
Outpatients with Psychosis (PICuP),
South London and Maudsley NHS
Foundation Trust, London, UK and
Institute of Psychiatry, Psychology and
Neuroscience, King's College London,
Department of Psychology, London UK

Araba Chintoh

Department of Psychiatry, University of
Toronto, Toronto, Canada

Christoph U. Correll

Hofstra Northwell School of Medicine,
Hempstead, New York, USA

John M. Davis

Department of Psychiatry, University of
Illinois Medical School, and John Hopkins
Medical School, Chicago and Baltimore,
USA

Siobhan Gee

National Psychosis Unit and Liaison
Psychiatry, South London and Maudsley
NHS Foundation Trust, London, UK

Oliver Howes

King's College London, London, Institute
of Medical Sciences (Imperial College
London) and Maudsley Hospital,
London, UK

Suzanne Jolley

Institute of Psychiatry, Psychology and
Neuroscience, King's College London,
London, UK and South London and
Maudsley NHS foundation trust,
London, UK

Stephen J. Kaar

Department of Psychosis Studies,
Institute of Psychiatry, Psychology and
Neuroscience, King's College London
and Maudsley Hospital, London UK

John Kane

Behavioral Health Services, Northwell
Health, New York, USA

Elizabeth Kuipers

Department of Psychology,
Institute of Psychiatry, Psychology and
Neuroscience, King's College London,
London, UK

John Lally

Department of Psychosis Studies,
Institute of Psychiatry, Psychology and
Neuroscience, King's College London,
London, UK

Jimmy Lee

Institute of Mental Health, Singapore;
Lee Kong Chian School of Medicine,
Nanyang Technological University,
Singapore

Stefan Leucht

Department of Psychiatry
and Psychotherapy, Technical
University of Munich, Munich,
Germany

James H. MacCabe

Department of Psychosis Studies,
Institute of Psychiatry, Psychology and
Neuroscience, King's College London,
London, UK

Stephen Marder

UCLA Psychiatry & Biobehavioral
Science, VA Greater LA Healthcare Sys,
Los Angeles, USA

Robert McCutcheon

Wellcome Trust, King's College London,
London, UK

Nobumi Miyake

Department of Neuropsychiatry,
St. Marianna University School of
Medicine, Miyamae-ku, Kawasaki,
Japan

Seiya Miyamoto

Department of Psychiatry,
Sakuragaoka Memorial Hospital,
Tokyo, Japan

Jimmi Nielsen

Mental Health Centre Glostrup, Mental
Health Services,Capital Region of
Denmark, University of Copenhagen,
Glostrup, Denmark

Juliana Onwumere

Department of Psychology,
Institute of Psychiatry, Psychology and
Neuroscience, King's College London,
London, UK

Emmanuelle Peters

Institute of Psychiatry, Psychology
and Neuroscience, King's College
London, London, UK and Psychological
Interventions Clinic for oupatients
with Psychosis (PICuP), South London
and Maudsley NHS foundation trust,
London, UK

Steven Potkin

Long Beach Veterans Administration
Health Care System, California, USA

Gary Remington

Department of Psychiatry, University of
Toronto, Toronto, Canada

Christopher Rohde

Mental Health Centre Glostrup, Mental
Health Services, Capital Region of
Denmark, University of Copenhagen,
Glostrup, Denmark

Robert C. Smith

Department of Psychiatry, New York
University School of Medicine and
Nathan Kline Institute for Psychiatric
Research, New York, USA

Hiroyoshi Takeuchi

Department of Neuropsychiatry,
Keio University School of Medicine,
Tokyo, Japan

David Taylor

Institute of Pharmaceutical Science,
King's College London, London, UK

Yvonne Yang

UCLA Psychiatry and Biobehavioral
Science/VA Greater Los Angeles
Healthcare System, Los Angeles, USA

CHAPTER 1

Introduction

Oliver Howes

KEY POINTS

- Schizophrenia and related psychotic disorders are common, affecting about 1 in 100 people.
- The treatment of schizophrenia is complex and, for most patients, needs to be sustained.
- A holistic approach to treatment is generally needed, encompassing drug treatments, as well as psychological, social, and family interventions.
- Treatment resistance is common and is a particular challenge both in its assessment and treatment.

Schizophrenia and related disorders are common, affecting about 1 in 100 people, and typically begin in late adolescence and early adulthood, when people are in the prime of their lives (Howes and Murray, 2014). They are also major causes of disease burden globally and are amongst the top causes of disability in working-age adults in the world (Whiteford et al., 2013). Carers are significantly affected by the burden of these disorders, which are a leading cause of healthcare costs (Wittchen et al., 2011). Schizophrenia and related disorders are also major causes of premature mortality due to suicide and elevated rates of comorbid conditions, particularly cardiometabolic disorders (Pillinger et al., 2017; Simon et al., 2018). It is clear that the stakes are high.

This highlights the importance of treating schizophrenia effectively. However, the treatment of schizophrenia is complex and, if it is to be done well, a challenge even to the most accomplished clinicians. Nevertheless, effective treatment of schizophrenia can transform lives for individuals and their carers.

This book considers the treatment of schizophrenia, with a particular focus on inadequate response and how to address it. It brings together contributions from leading, clinically orientated, experts from a variety of backgrounds across the world. These contributions cover treatment of the first episode and maintaining response, as well as the principles underlying determining treatment response and resistance, the neurobiology underlying them, and the epidemiology of treatment resistance.

Clozapine remains the only licensed drug treatment for treatment-resistant schizophrenia. However, it is a challenging treatment to implement and use effectively. The book covers the fundamental aspects of using clozapine, before addressing its complexities in chapters devoted to managing its side effects and using it in special cases. Clozapine is not suitable for many treatment-resistant patients and alternatives to clozapine are considered. Moreover, clozapine is not effective in all patients. The book also considers drug and other treatment options in this case. Effective treatment for schizophrenia requires more than drug treatment alone. Family therapy and cognitive behavioural approaches are discussed by leading practitioners, who have pioneered their development and application to schizophrenia and particularly treatment resistance. Electroconvulsive therapy and other treatments are discussed and their role in treatment considered. The book is intended to be clinically focused and to help clinicians and students to think about how to help their patients. With this in mind, there is a chapter of representative case studies drawn from the collective clinical experience of all the authors to illustrate the principles and application of the evidence discussed in the book.

There is a strong emphasis throughout the book on the latest and most robust evidence, particularly that derived from randomized, double-blind controlled trials and meta-analyses where this is available. However, clinical practice is rarely as clear-cut as the protocol for a trial, and patients do not often conform to the strict inclusion criteria that trials require. Moreover, in many instances evidence from randomized, double-blind controlled trials is not available. Indeed, it may not be feasible or ethical for such a trial to be conducted. This means that other forms of evidence need to be drawn on and the evidence interpreted and applied judiciously to help the individual patient. The authors do this, indicating where this is the case so that the reader can appraise the evidence in light of its limitations.

Collectively the authors have well over half a millennium's worth of experience in treating patients with schizophrenia and related disorders. They have drawn on this, as well as the latest research, to provide a framework to help clinicians and researchers interpret and apply the evidence to treat schizophrenia.

It is clear throughout the book that there are unmet treatment needs in schizophrenia. The final chapter focuses on where the field is going, considering new and emerging treatments. A number of trials and other studies are currently under way that could revolutionize the treatment of schizophrenia and particularly treatment resistance. This chapter discusses the most promising new strategies and how far they have progressed so that the reader may appreciate what is on the horizon.

The stakes are high when treating schizophrenia. This book aims to help the clinician give their patients the best odds of getting better, and researchers, students, and other readers a thorough understanding of the clinical challenges and the latest evidence on how to approach them.

REFERENCES

Howes, O. D., Murray, R. M. (2014). Schizophrenia: an integrated sociodevelopmental-cognitive model. *Lancet*, 383, 1677–87.

Pillinger, T., Beck, K., Gobjila, C., Donocik, J. G., Jauhar, S., Howes, O. D. (2017). Impaired glucose homeostasis in first-episode schizophrenia: a systematic review and meta-analysis. *JAMA Psychiatry*, 74, 261–9.

Simon, G. E., Stewart, C., Yarborough, B. J., et al. (2018). Mortality rates after the first diagnosis of psychotic disorder in adolescents and young adults. *JAMA Psychiatry*, 75, 254–60.

Whiteford, H. A., Degenhardt, L., Rehm, J., et al. (2013). Global burden of disease attributable to mental and substance use disorders: findings from the Global Burden of Disease Study 2010. *Lancet*, 382, 1575–86.

Wittchen, H. U., Jacobi, F., Rehm, J., et al. (2011). The size and burden of mental disorders and other disorders of the brain in Europe 2010. *Eur Neuropsychopharmacol*, 21, 655–79.

CHAPTER 2

Treatment response and resistance in schizophrenia: principles and definitions

Robert McCutcheon, Christoph U. Correll, Oliver Howes, and John Kane

---

KEY POINTS

- The criteria that have been used to define treatment response and treatment resistance vary, and this needs to be considered when comparing studies.
- A consensus approach has recently been developed to address this.
- The use of standardized rating scales is recommended to evaluate response and resistance where possible, and particularly when using third-line interventions.
- At least a 50% reduction in symptom severity ratings (25% in resistant patients) is considered clinically meaningful.
- Only 5% of clinical trials of drugs for treatment resistance used the same definition of treatment resistance and treatment intolerance.
- The concept of treatment resistance includes adequate duration, dose, and adherence to treatment coupled with persistent symptoms and functional impairment.
- The diagnosis should be reviewed and pseudoresistance ruled out as part of the evaluation of treatment resistance.

Treatment response

Schizophrenia shows a range of responses to treatment, both in terms of absolute symptom change and the time course to change (Kapur et al., 2000; Kinon et al., 2010; Marques et al., 2011). Notwithstanding this, the categorical classification of response is useful both in clinical and research settings where binary decisions, such as which treatment to choose, have to be made. A number of different criteria have been used to define treatment response, including relatively small percentage reductions in symptom ratings that may not be clinically meaningful (Leucht et al., 2009). Reflecting a focus on clinically meaningful change, it has been proposed that at least a 50% reduction in symptom scores should be observed to classify an individual as a 'responder' in trials of acutely ill patients whose condition is not thought to be treatment-resistant, and that in trials of resistant patients, this threshold could be relaxed to 25% (Leucht et al., 2009; Leucht, 2014). Whilst these cut-offs are useful as clinically meaningful endpoints, it is preferable if studies report additional detail on symptom change, including the percentage of responders using other cut-offs (e.g. <0%, 1–24%, 25–49%, 50–74%, and 75–100% improvement) as well, to facilitate comparison between studies and inform clinical decision-making (Leucht, 2014). The Treatment Response and Resistance in Psychosis (TRRIP) working group suggested a complementary definition of response for use in settings where a prospective trial of treatment had not occurred, proposing that responders could be classified cross-sectionally as those individuals showing no more than mild symptom severity across the symptom items in the domain(s) of interest, consistently for at least 12 weeks (Howes et al., 2017).

One important issue is that many of the rating scales commonly used to index symptom severity have minimum scores (i.e. even a volunteer with no health problems will score more than zero). This means that a percentage change in symptom severity that is calculated without adjusting for the minimum score is biased. Thus, regardless of the rating scale used, it is important that the scale is zero floored when calculating percentage change in symptom severity to avoid bias (e.g. in the case of the Positive And Negative Syndrome Scale, 30 points should be subtracted from total scores before percentage change is calculated) (Obermeier et al., 2010). Surprisingly, this has not always been recognized, and many studies report percentage change without adjusting for the minimum score (Obermeier et al., 2011).

The related concept of remission refers to remaining free of clinically significant symptoms for an extended period. The Schizophrenia Working Group proposed that, to meet remission criteria, an individual should have a severity score of mild or less for at least 6 months for the following symptoms: delusions, hallucinations, disorganized speech, disorganized behaviour, and negative symptoms (Andreasen et al., 2005). Whilst these criteria did not explicitly define a minimum level of functioning, the proposed definition for 'mild' severity means, by definition, that symptoms do not interfere significantly with day-to-day functioning. Recovery refers to the regaining of social and occupational functioning and a return to the premorbid state (Leucht, 2014). This is separate to the 'personal recovery' concept that has developed in service user movements, where 'recovery' places more weight upon self-reported patient experiences and does not necessarily reflect the clinician's viewpoint (Leamy et al., 2011). However, neither concept of functional nor personal recovery has widely accepted, operationalized criteria to date and, partly as a result, they are less frequently used as trial outcomes than change in symptoms or remission.

Varying definitions of resistance

Soon after the introduction of dopamine antagonists for the treatment of schizophrenia in the 1950s it was apparent that, while these were effective treatments for many patients, there was a sizeable proportion of individuals who derived little benefit from these drugs. However, it was the subsequent demonstration by Kane et al. (1988) that clozapine was of particular effectiveness in these patients that crystallized the concept of treatment-resistant schizophrenia (TRS). The precise definition of this concept has, however, varied considerably since then.

To be classified as treatment-resistant in the original Kane trial of clozapine, participants needed to fulfil the following criteria: (1) at least three periods of treatment in the past 5 years with antipsychotics from different chemical classes, at dosages above 1000 mg chlorpromazine equivalents; (2) no period of good functioning in the past 5 years; (3) a Brief Psychiatric Rating Scale (BPRS) score of ≥45 with at least moderate scores on two of the positive symptom items *and* a clinical global impression severity score of ≥4; and then (4) complete a prospective 6-week trial of haloperidol without significant improvement in symptoms.

Inclusion criteria for subsequent clinical trials in TRS have typically been less stringent than these. For the most part they have included the core concept that individuals must have received adequate pharmacological treatment, and that significant symptoms have persisted despite this treatment, but precise definitions vary significantly.

A recent systematic review of definitions of TRS used in clinical trials identified 42 eligible studies (Howes et al., 2017). A summary of findings is shown in Fig. 2.1. This shows that, of the 42 trials, only 50% reported operationalized criteria that included the use of a standardized rating scale, specified minimum symptom duration, and specified adequate prior treatment in terms of minimum dosage, duration, and number of previous antipsychotics. The other studies often give limited detail and rely on local clinicians to identify patients as treatment-resistant based on their own judgement and practice, which could be affected by multiple factors such as referral biases and differences in clinical settings (patients in long-term inpatient settings may be very different to those in community teams, for example). Thus, there is a problem for interpreting and applying the findings from the studies that did not use operationalized criteria. Furthermore, only two of the studies (5%) used identical criteria, highlighting that, even where operationalized criteria were used, there was variability. It is also important to note that some of the studies included treatment-intolerant patients as well as individuals whose illness was treatment-resistant. In terms of the most commonly used definitions: 62% of studies required a minimum of two previous antipsychotic treatment periods, 57% defined adequate duration as a minimum of 6 weeks, and 38% used a prospective phase of supervised treatment. However, it is striking, given the high rates of poor antipsychotic adherence reported in studies of people with persistent psychotic symptoms, i.e. 35% have been shown to have subtherapeutic or zero antipsychotic blood levels (McCutcheon et al., 2018), that none of the studies operationalized the assessment of past adherence to antipsychotic treatment.

The use of inconsistent criteria across studies means that it is difficult to compare findings across studies, whether this be in clinical trials or in neuroimaging,

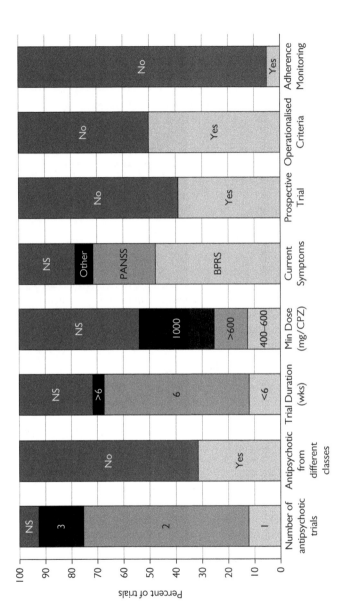

Fig. 2.1 Summary of criteria used in published clinical trials of treatment-resistant schizophrenia. This shows that there is considerable variation in reporting between trials and that the criteria that are used to define treatment resistance vary considerably. CPZ = chlorpromazine equivalent dose.

epidemiological, or genetic studies of treatment resistance. This problem likely contributes to the high degree of heterogeneity seen in both clinical and neuroimaging studies (Mouchlianitis et al., 2016; Samara et al., 2016; Siskind et al., 2016). This issue of inconsistent or absent criteria for TRS in many studies may further partially account for some inconsistencies between the findings of different clinical trials (e.g. Bitter et al., 2004; Buchanan et al., 2005), as the individuals included in one trial may be quite different from those included in another, despite both being reported as trials of TRS. For example, the study by Bitter et al. included those with only one failed past trial of an antipsychotic for 4 weeks, considered intolerability to be equivalent to resistance, and found olanzapine to be efficacious, while the study by Buchanan et al. required individuals to have had two previous antipsychotic trials of 6 weeks, and an additional prospective trial, and found no benefit with the same drug.

The consensus definition of treatment-resistant schizophrenia and underlying principles

To address the heterogeneity in definitions of treatment resistance, the TRRIP working group was formed to establish consensus, standardized criteria for the diagnosis of TRS. Over 50 experts in the field developed the criteria following the results of a systematic review of existing definitions, online surveys, and multiple meetings to discuss issues and achieve a consensus. The consensus criteria that were developed are discussed in the following sections and are summarized in Table 2.1.

Terminology and exclusion of other causes

It is recommended that the term 'treatment-resistant schizophrenia' be consistently used in preference to alternatives to enable efficient searching for relevant studies.

All patients should have a diagnosis of schizophrenia confirmed using established criteria and a clinical review to confirm that their symptoms are not secondary to other causes such as substance use. Care should be taken to ensure that all physical and psychiatric comorbidities are appropriately treated, and that current psychotic symptoms are not secondary to these.

Clinical characteristics

The following clinical characteristics and approaches to assessment were identified by the TRRIP working group. These are designed to reflect the principle that treatment resistance identifies a group of patients with clinically significant, persistent illness. This aims to distinguish treatment resistance from a short-lived worsening in symptoms, for example secondary to an acute stress, or a mild illness that may not warrant potentially risky or invasive interventions.

Table 2.1 Consensus criteria for assessment and definition of treatment-resistant schizophrenia

Domain	Subdomain	Minimum requirement	Optimum requirement
Current symptoms	Assessment	Interview using standardized rating scale (e.g. PANSS, BPRS, SANS, SAPS)	Prospective evaluation of treatment using standardized rating scale
	Severity	At least moderate severity	At least moderate severity and <20% symptom reduction during prospective trial/observation ≥6 weeks
	Duration	≥12 weeks	≥12 weeks. Specify duration of treatment resistance
	Subjective distress	Not required	Not required
	Functioning	At least moderate functional impairment measured using a validated scale (e.g. SOFAS)	At least moderate functional impairment measured using a validated scale (e.g. SOFAS)
Adequate treatment	Assessment of past response	Information to be gathered from patient/carer reports, staff and case notes, pill counts, and dispensing charts	Information to be gathered from patient/carer reports, staff and case notes, pill counts, and dispensing charts
	Duration	≥6 weeks at a therapeutic dose. Record minimum and mean (SD) duration for each treatment episode	≥6 weeks at a therapeutic dose. Record minimum and mean (SD) duration for each treatment episode
	Dose	Equivalent to ≥600 mg chlorpromazine per day.[1] Record minimum and mean (SD) dose for each drug	Equivalent to ≥600 mg chlorpromazine per day.[1] Record minimum and mean (SD) dose for each drug
	Number of antipsychotics	≥2 past adequate treatment episodes with different antipsychotic drugs Specify median number of failed antipsychotic trials	≥2 past treatment episodes with different antipsychotic drugs and at least one utilizing a long-acting injectable antipsychotic (for at least 4 months). Specify median number of failed antipsychotic trials

continued >

Table 2.1 Consensus criteria for assessment and definition of treatment-resistant schizophrenia *(continued)*

Domain	Subdomain	Minimum requirement	Optimum requirement
	Current adherence	≥80% of prescribed doses taken. Adherence should be assessed using ≥2 of pill counts, dispensing chart reviews, and patient/carer report. Antipsychotic plasma levels monitored on at least one occasion Specify methods used to establish adherence	As for minimum criteria and additionally trough antipsychotic serum levels measured on at least two occasions separated by at least 2 weeks (without prior notification of patient)
Symptom domain		Positive/negative/cognitive	
Time course		Early-onset (within 1 year of treatment onset)/ medium-term onset (within >1–5 years of treatment onset)/late-onset (after >5 years of treatment onset)	
Ultra-treatment-resistant: clozapine		Meets the criteria for treatment resistance plus failure to respond to adequate clozapine treatment	

BPRS, Brief Psychiatric Rating Scale; PANSS, Positive And Negative Syndrome Scale; SANS, Scale for the Assessment of Negative Symptoms; SAPS, Scale for the Assessment of Positive Symptoms; SD, standard deviation; SOFAS, Social and Occupational Functioning Scale.

[1] Based on established conversion criteria (e.g. Gardner et al., 2010; Leucht et al., 2014; 2015).

Rating scales

A validated symptom rating scale should be used to assess symptoms so that it is clear how they were assessed and to ensure that symptoms are measured in a reliable and standardized way. Examples include the Positive And Negative Syndrome Scale (PANSS), Brief Psychiatric Rating Scale (BPRS), Scale for the Assessment of Negative Symptoms (SANS), or Scale for the Assessment of Positive Symptoms (SAPS) (Overall and Gorham, 1962; Andreasen, 1984a; 1984b; Kay et al., 1987).

Absolute thresholds

Symptoms should be of at least moderate severity for at least two symptoms in each domain under study. If only one symptom is present, it should be at least severe. Symptoms should have been present at this severity for a minimum of 12 weeks.

Symptom change with treatment

In addition to absolute thresholds, the response to treatment must be established. This should ideally be undertaken prospectively, and only individuals whose illness has shown <20% improvement on a standardized rating scale following treatment and where the symptom ratings still fulfil the absolute threshold should be categorized as treatment-resistant. If retrospective assessment is used, then as much collateral information as possible should be obtained to support decisions and, during past treatment episodes, patients should have been rated as less than 'minimally improved' on the Clinical Global Impression-Schizophrenia Scale (Haro et al., 2003).

Functional impact

Functional impact should also be measured with a validated rating scale such as the Social and Occupational Functioning Scale (SOFAS) (Morosini et al., 2000) and should be of moderate or greater severity.

Adequate treatment

These criteria were developed to reflect the principle that patients have received treatment in a form that would generally be expected to result in a response and to exclude suboptimally treated patients.

Duration

Each antipsychotic treatment episode should have lasted for a minimum of 6 weeks. Ideally at least one treatment episode should consist of a long-acting injectable antipsychotic formulation to ensure that non-response is not secondary to poor or inadequate adherence.

Dosage

The minimum dosage should be either the target dose or, where there is a range, the midpoint of the target range as given in the manufacturer's summary of product characteristics. If this is not possible then a total daily dose equivalent of 600 mg chlorpromazine should be used, calculated using published criteria such as those described by Leucht and colleagues (2014; 2015). An exception may be made for patients with first-episode schizophrenia with primary treatment resistance or paediatric patients with early-onset schizophrenia who are often more sensitive to adverse effects of antipsychotics and who may not tolerate doses of up to 600 mg chlorpromazine equivalent. If a trial is aborted owing to medication intolerance before an individual has been treated at an adequate dose for 6 weeks, it should not be considered an adequate trial.

Number of treatment episodes

A minimum of two failed treatment trials meeting the criteria discussed in the section on 'Dosage' is required to establish treatment resistance. Ideally, one of these should consist of a trial of a long-acting injectable antipsychotic.

Adherence

It is important to identify when a lack of response is secondary to medication ineffectiveness as opposed to inadequate levels due to non-adherence

(McCutcheon et al., 2015). Patients should have taken ≥80% of prescribed doses for at least ≥12 weeks. This should be determined using as many sources as possible: patient and carer reports, pharmacy records, pill counts. In addition, it is recommended that antipsychotic plasma levels should be checked without notice on at least one and, preferably, on at least two occasions in all patients taking oral antipsychotics. If possible, a period of guaranteed adherence should be ensured using a long-acting injectable or a period of directly monitored treatment.

Subspecifiers

These criteria were developed to reflect the principle that symptom domains may not all be equally resistant to treatment, and that there may be important differences in the clinical course of treatment resistance. They are intended to help clarity in description and facilitate research.

Clinical

The primary symptom domain affecting individuals should be recorded as positive, negative, or cognitive. Individuals may meet criteria for multiple domains, e.g. 'treatment-resistant schizophrenia, positive and negative domains'.

Degree

While treatment resistance is frequently treated as a binary concept, there is a spectrum of severity, and symptom scores should be recorded and reported whenever possible to facilitate comparison.

Temporal development

In some cases, resistance to antipsychotic treatment is apparent from illness onset, whereas in other cases resistance is something that develops after an initial response to treatment. To allow for research into the clinical and biological differences between these two situations it is recommended that a subspecifier of early-onset (within the first year of treatment), medium term-onset (between >1 and 5 years), or late-onset (more than 5 years after initial treatment) be used where possible.

Clozapine resistance

If an individual has failed to respond to clozapine this should be classified as 'ultra-medication treatment-resistant schizophrenia' or 'clozapine-resistant schizophrenia'. To be classified as having a clozapine-resistant illness, individuals should have been treated with a dose at least in the midpoint of the therapeutic range, but in addition should have evidence of clozapine plasma levels at least ≥350 ng/mL on *at least* two separate occasions, and treatment should have lasted for *at least* 3 months following the attainment of a therapeutic plasma level.

The criteria outlined are not a significant departure from existing definitions. The primary difference is that these consensus criteria operationalize core aspects of the definition, including the nature and severity of ongoing symptoms and an adequate treatment episode. The adoption of these criteria and their use as benchmarks for reporting should help to ensure that it is easier to compare future research studies.

Implications for clinical practice

The findings from the systematic review discussed indicate that there has been considerable variation in definitions of treatment resistance (Howes et al., 2017), with only 5% of studies using the same definitions and some studies mixing treatment intolerance with treatment resistance. These findings have a number of important implications for clinical practice. Firstly, they indicate that it is important to check that the characteristics of the patients recruited into a trial are representative of the patient in front of you before using the evidence to inform practice. Secondly, the different inclusion criteria used, such as including intolerant patients in some studies, means that in certain cases it is not possible to compare trials. These design differences between studies need to be considered in meta-analyses to avoid potential bias. Finally, they highlight the potential value of a systematic approach to assessing treatment resistance in clinical practice.

The criteria for treatment resistance developed by the TRRIP working group are not intended to be applied to routine clinical practice or to restrict clinical practice. However, the criteria (see Table 2.1) are intended to inform clinical practice and to be a useful guide to the clinical assessment of patients, albeit that not all aspects of the recommended assessment will routinely be possible. Nevertheless, this approach has been employed in routine clinical practice, indicating that it is feasible (Beck et al., 2014). The assessment of adequate treatment is a particularly important component of the work-up that it is worth focusing on in clinical practice, given findings that in typical clinical populations a significant proportion of those suspected to have treatment resistance have not received adequate treatment (McCutcheon et al., 2018). It can also be useful to use prospective trials of treatment, and include symptom ratings, to help to determine treatment resistance and to evaluate the benefit of treatment.

Conclusions

A striking degree of variability in the definitions of treatment response and resistance has been used in studies, which makes comparisons across studies difficult, and could explain inconsistencies in some findings. This needs to be borne in mind when reviewing the literature and applying it to clinical practice. Moreover, many studies have not reported clear definitions and/or evaluated key components of treatment resistance. Recent proposals aim to address these limitations by providing operationalized criteria. Whilst these are not intended to be used in routine clinical practice, the principles are applicable to the clinical assessment of a patient who may be treatment-resistant. The core component of treatment response is a clinically meaningful improvement that is readily observed in routine clinical practice without recourse to structured clinical rating scales. The key aspect of treatment resistance is the presence of persistent, clinically significant symptoms despite adequate treatment. Studies indicate that some patients are mistakenly thought to be treatment-resistant when they have not received adequate treatment (tolerated dose, blood level duration), highlighting the importance of assessing the adequacy of treatment, including using objective measures, such as measuring plasma antipsychotic levels where possible, and using long-acting injectable formulations of antipsychotics before declaring someone treatment-resistant.

REFERENCES

Andreasen, N. C. (1984a). *Scale for the Assessment of Negative Symptoms*. Iowa City: University of Iowa.

Andreasen, N. C. (1984b). *Scale for the Assessment of Positive Symptoms*. Iowa City: University of Iowa.

Andreasen, N. C., Carpenter, W. T., Kane, J. M., Lasser, R. A., Marder, S. R., Weinberger, D. R. (2005). Remission in schizophrenia: proposed criteria and rationale for consensus. *Am J Psychiatry*, 162, 441–9.

Beck, K., McCutcheon, R., Bloomfield, M. A. P., et al. (2014). The practical management of refractory schizophrenia—the Maudsley Treatment Review and Assessment Team service approach. *Acta Psychiatr Scand*, 130, 427–38.

Bitter, I., Dossenbach, M. R. K., Brook, S., et al. (2004). Olanzapine versus clozapine in treatment-resistant or treatment-intolerant schizophrenia. *Prog Neuro-Psychopharmacology Biol Psychiatry*, 28, 173–80.

Buchanan, R. W., Ball, M. P., Weiner, E., et al. (2005). Olanzapine treatment of residual positive and negative symptoms. *Am J Psychiatry*, 162, 124–9.

Gardner, D. M., Murphy, A. L., O'Donnell, H., Centorrino, F., Baldessarini, R. J. (2010). International consensus study of antipsychotic dosing. *Am J Psychiatry*, 167, 686–93.

Haro, J. M., Kamath, S. A., Ochoa, S., et al. (2003). The Clinical Global Impression-Schizophrenia scale: a simple instrument to measure the diversity of symptoms present in schizophrenia. *Acta Psychiatr Scand Suppl*, 107, 16–23.

Howes, O. D., McCutcheon, R., Agid, O., et al. (2017), Treatment-resistant schizophrenia: Treatment Response and Resistance in Psychosis (TRRIP) Working Group Consensus Guidelines on Diagnosis and Terminology. *Am J Psychiatry*, 174, 216–29.

Kane, J., Honigfeld, G., Singer, J., Meltzer, H. (1988). Clozapine for the treatment-resistant schizophrenic. A double-blind comparison with chlorpromazine. *Arch Gen Psych*, 45, 789–96.

Kapur, S., Zipursky, R., Jones, C., Remington, G., Houle, S. (2000). Relationship between dopamine D(2) occupancy, clinical response, and side effects: a double-blind PET study of first-episode schizophrenia. *Am J Psychiatry*, 157, 514–20.

Kay, S. R., Flszbein, A., Opler, L. A. (1987). The Positive And Negative Syndrome Scale for Schizophrenia. *Schizophr Bull*, 13, 261–76.

Kinon, B. J., Chen, L., Ascher-Svanum, H., et al. (2010). Early response to antipsychotic drug therapy as a clinical marker of subsequent response in the treatment of schizophrenia. *Neuropsychopharmacology*, 35, 581–90.

Leamy, M., Bird, V., Le Boutillier, C., Williams, J., Slade, M. (2011). Conceptual framework for personal recovery in mental health: systematic review and narrative synthesis. *Br J Psychiatry*, 199, 445–52.

Leucht, S. (2014). Measurements of response, remission, and recovery in schizophrenia and examples for their clinical application. *J Clin Psychiatry*, 75 (Suppl. 1), 8–14.

Leucht, S., Davis, J. M., Engel, R. R., Kissling, W., Kane, J. M. (2009). Definitions of response and remission in schizophrenia: recommendations for their use and their presentation. *Acta Psychiatr Scand*, 119, 7–14.

Leucht, S., Samara, M., Heres, S., et al. (2015). Dose equivalents for second-generation antipsychotic drugs: the classical mean dose method. *Schizophr Bull*, 41, 1397–1402.

Leucht, S., Samara, M., Heres, S., Patel, M. X., Woods, S. W., Davis, J. M. (2014). Dose equivalents for second-generation antipsychotics: the minimum effective dose method. *Schizophr Bull*, 40, 314–26.

Marques, T. R., Arenovich, T., Agid, O., et al. (2011). The different trajectories of antipsychotic response: antipsychotics versus placebo. *Psychol Med*, 41, 1481–8.

McCutcheon, R., Beck, K., Bloomfield, M. A. P., et al. (2015). Treatment resistant or resistant to treatment? Antipsychotic plasma levels in patients with poorly controlled psychotic symptoms. *J Psychopharmacol*, 29, 892–7.

McCutcheon, R., Beck, K., D'Ambrosio, E., et al. (2018). Antipsychotic plasma levels in the assessment of poor treatment response in schizophrenia. *Acta Psychiatr Scand*, 137, 39–46.

Morosini, P. L., Magliano, L., Brambilla, L., Ugolini, S., Pioli, R. (2000). Development, reliability and acceptability of a new version of the DSM-IV Social and Occupational Functioning Assessment Scale (SOFAS) to assess routine social functioning. *Acta Psychiatr Scand*, 101, 323–9.

Mouchlianitis, E., McCutcheon, R., Howes, O. D. (2016). Brain-imaging studies of treatment-resistant schizophrenia: a systematic review. *The Lancet Psychiatry*, 366, 1–13.

Obermeier, M., Mayr, A., Schennach-Wolff, R., Seemu, F. (2010). Should the PANSS be rescaled? *Schizophr Bull*, 36, 455–60.

Obermeier, M., Schennach-Wolff, R., Meyer, S., et al. (2011). Is the PANSS used correctly? A systematic review. *BMC Psychiatry*, 11, 113.

Overall, J. E., Gorham, D. O. R. (1962). The Brief Psychiatric Rating Scale. *Psychol Rep*, 10, 799–812.

Samara, M. T., Dold, M., Gianatsi, M., et al. (2016). efficacy, acceptability, and tolerability of antipsychotics in treatment-resistant schizophrenia. *JAMA Psychiatry*, 73, 199–210.

Siskind, D., McCartney, L., Goldschlager, R., Kisely, S. (2016). Clozapine v. first- and second-generation antipsychotics in treatment-refractory schizophrenia: systematic review and meta-analysis. *Br J Psychiatry*, 209, 385–92.

Maximizing response to first-line antipsychotics in schizophrenia

Robert C. Smith, Stefan Leucht, and John M. Davis

KEY POINTS

- The choice of first-line antipsychotic treatment for patients with schizophrenia should balance considerations of differential efficacy of antipsychotics against the relative risk of different side effects.

- Recent meta-analyses have shown that antipsychotics are not equivalent in efficacy. Clozapine, amisulpride, olanzapine, and risperidone show small to moderate, but statistically significant, differences, indicating greater efficacy compared to a number of other antipsychotics on some primary efficacy outcome measures.

- Amisulpride and cariprazine have the strongest evidence for greater efficacy for treating negative symptoms relative to other antipsychotics.

- Clozapine and olanzapine have among the highest weight gain potential and amisulpride has more effects on QTc prolongation and prolactin elevation than other commonly used antipsychotics.

- There is little evidence to support using doses above the therapeutic range other than in exceptional circumstances.

Introduction

Before concluding that patients with schizophrenia are truly treatment-resistant we should consider whether they have shown maximal response to first-line treatment. This requires evaluation as to whether patients have been treated with the most efficacious antipsychotic in light of the tolerability of the drug's side effects, whether they have been treated with adequate doses of the most appropriate first-line antipsychotic, and whether response could be further maximized by adding an adjunctive medication or switching to another first-line antipsychotic. There are now many antipsychotics available for the clinician to choose from for first-line treatment of a patient with schizophrenia. Almost all these drugs have evidence for greater efficacy than placebo. Some earlier studies, however, have suggested that there may be little or no difference in efficacy of different antipsychotics when used at an appropriate dose. The CATIE study, published more than 10 years ago (Lieberman et al., 2005), showed little difference in overall efficacy between three second-generation antipsychotics and a first-generation antipsychotic (perphenazine). However, on some measures, time to discontinuation for any cause and decrease in Positive and Negative Syndrome Scale (PANSS) scores at 6 months, olanzapine appeared slightly superior to some of the other antipsychotics. In this chapter, we review evidence that has accumulated during the past 15 years, primarily from statistical analysis of controlled studies using meta-analysis techniques. From these studies we summarize the differential efficacy and side effects of antipsychotics, and how these differences might inform clinical decisions on preferential drugs for first-line treatment of schizophrenia. This review concentrates on results of studies of standard treatment for acute episodes of schizophrenia, whether for first episode or relapsing patients. It does not deal in depth with studies specifically examining patients with treatment-resistant schizophrenia, patients with only prodromal symptoms, or with maintenance treatment of schizophrenia after resolution of acute symptoms.

Review of the evidence for efficacy

Methodological approaches

We believe that recent systematic reviews using meta-analysis techniques have provided convincing evidence for differences in efficacy among different antipsychotics, although the magnitude of differences in most of the comparisons is not large. These studies have used both pair-wise meta-analysis, which compares multiple studies in which two specific drugs or drug and placebo were evaluated in the same study, and network meta-analysis (Table 3.1), a new statistical technique that allows comparison of drugs from different studies if some statistical characteristics (in particular, transitivity) of the data are met. The advantage of network meta-analysis is that it often allows comparison of efficacy of two antipsychotics from a considerably larger number of studies and therefore it sometimes produces new or more robust findings than can be obtained for pair-wise meta-analysis (Leucht et al., 2016a). Meta-analysis provides more reliable estimates of comparative efficacy than reviews that are based on interpretations of the literature or 'counting' of positive results because: a) it is based on statistical estimates from multiple studies using standard statistical transformation of original data; b) it allows assessment of statistically significant effects in overall studies, although some of the individual studies may have had too small a sample or too large variation to produce a statistically significant difference between drugs for that specific study; c) it allows statistical analysis of the ways in which many factors in the design of included studies can potentially affect summary outcome results; and d) it provides a standard for evaluating the extent of various bias factors in study design in the sample of studies chosen for analysis, which may have a potential influence on the validity of the conclusions and/or the confidence in the overall results (Higgins and Green, 2008; Borenstein et al., 2009).

Table 3.1 Comparison of pair-wise and network meta-analyses

Conventional, pair-wise, meta-analysis	Network (multiple treatments) meta-analysis
Uses data where two treatments were investigated in the same trial—*direct comparisons*	Uses data from *direct comparisons* as in pair-wise meta-analysis as well as data from *indirect comparisons* if this can be validly estimated. For example, indirect comparison of efficacy of drug A versus drug C when there are only studies of drug A versus drug B and drug B versus drug C
Compares relative efficacy of two specific treatments, and gives effect size of difference between the two treatments from multiple studies. It cannot provide a statistical metric for comparison between different pairs of drugs	Can rank multiple treatments in terms of efficacy or other criteria and can give effect size differences between multiple treatments
	In network meta-analysis it is important to assess degree of transitivity in the network, i.e. the extent to which potential effect modifiers are similarly operative in all the compared trials

Efficacy of antipsychotic drugs

Differences in overall efficacy

A recent comprehensive network meta-analysis study of 15 different antipsychotic drugs (Leucht et al., 2013) found clozapine more efficacious in measures of overall efficacy than most other antipsychotic drugs, with differences in effect sizes ranging from small (standard mean difference [SMD] 0.2–0.33) to moderate (0.40–0.55) in comparison with the other antipsychotics. Amisulpride, olanzapine, and risperidone showed relatively small increases in efficacy (SMD 0.11–0.33) compared to haloperidol and some other more recent, second-generation antipsychotics (SGAs) (Fig. 3.1). However, all the antipsychotics were more efficacious than placebo, with effect size ranging from small (0.33) for iloperidone to large (0.88) for clozapine, and this overall efficacy was further confirmed in a pair-wise meta-analysis of all placebo-controlled studies (Leucht et al., 2013; 2017). Since the overall effect sizes of efficacy between drug and placebo were generally not more than small to moderate in size, the relatively smaller differences in greater efficacy for amisulpride, olanzapine, and risperidone compared to some other first- and second-generation antipsychotics may be clinically meaningful. The higher effect size of the clozapine in comparison with other antipsychotics in the network meta-analysis may be partially explained by the fact that the clozapine comparisons to other drugs were

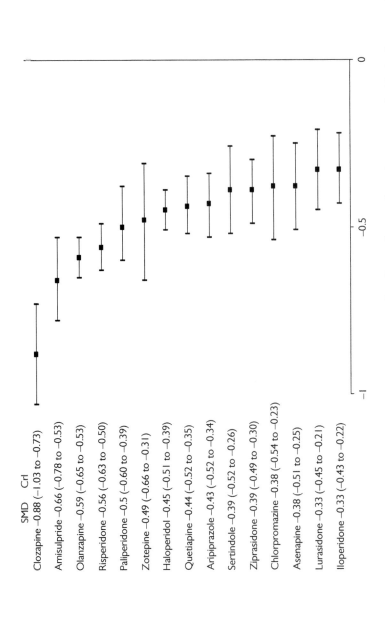

	SMD	CrI
Clozapine	−0.88	(−1.03 to −0.73)
Amisulpride	−0.66	(−0.78 to −0.53)
Olanzapine	−0.59	(−0.65 to −0.53)
Risperidone	−0.56	(−0.63 to −0.50)
Paliperidone	−0.5	(−0.60 to −0.39)
Zotepine	−0.49	(−0.66 to −0.31)
Haloperidol	−0.45	(−0.51 to −0.39)
Quetiapine	−0.44	(−0.52 to −0.35)
Aripiprazole	−0.43	(−0.52 to −0.34)
Sertindole	−0.39	(−0.52 to −0.26)
Ziprasidone	−0.39	(−0.49 to −0.30)
Chlorpromazine	−0.38	(−0.54 to −0.23)
Asenapine	−0.38	(−0.51 to −0.25)
Lurasidone	−0.33	(−0.45 to −0.21)
Iloperidone	−0.33	(−0.43 to −0.22)

Fig. 3.1 Differences in overall efficacy of antipsychotic drugs. Forest plot for efficacy of antipsychotic drugs compared with placebo, network meta-analysis. Treatments are ranked according to their surface under the cumulative ranking (SUCRA) values. SMD = standardized mean difference. CrI = credible interval.

Reprinted from *The Lancet*, 14, 382, Leucht S., Cipriani A., Spineli L. et al, Comparative efficacy and tolerability of 15 antipsychotic drugs in schizophrenia: a multiple-treatments meta-analysis, pp. 951–92. Copyright (2013) with permission from Elsevier.

mainly based on older clozapine studies with first-generation antipsychotics (FGAs), and these statistically significant differences were not replicated when direct comparisons were made between clozapine and SGAs tested in the same study, when we used pair-wise meta-analysis. Although the magnitude of drug versus placebo differences in antipsychotic studies of efficacy has decreased over time, a recent analysis of all placebo-controlled studies (Fig. 3.2) (Leucht et al., 2017) clearly shows that this is not because of the decreased response rate or improvement in the antipsychotic drugs but primarily because of the increased placebo response rate over the years.

It is important to note that, although there were some important efficacy differences among the antipsychotics, the primary measure in most meta-analyses was mean response difference for any validated response measure; this approach does not separate drugs that could produce a good clinical response (e.g. 50% improvement in symptoms) from drugs that produced a minimal response (e.g. 20%). Leucht and associates (2017) have shown that there is a much larger difference between drug versus placebo when any (minimal) response (50% drug versus 30% placebo) is measured than when drugs are compared using measures that indicate much improvement or a 'good' response (23% drug versus 14% placebo). This degree of difference in response between drug and placebo contrasts with the large improvement seen in antipsychotic drug efficacy in the early National Institute of Mental Health studies (61% improvement in symptoms under drug compared to only 23% under placebo) (Guttmacher, 1964). However, these early studies were mostly done in first-episode patients, whereas most of the modern meta-analyses have relied on studies done with multi-episode schizophrenic patients. Whether there are differences among antipsychotic drugs in the proportion of patients who show a good clinical response (e.g. greater than 50% reduction in symptoms) has not been explored as systematically in meta-analysis studies.

Differential efficacy for types of symptoms or stage of illness

Are there differences in efficacy for types of symptoms or stage of illness among antipsychotic drugs?

Positive symptoms

Studies using pair-wise meta-analysis comparisons indicate that amisulpride, olanzapine, clozapine, and risperidone are more efficacious than FGAs in reducing positive symptoms. There were few differences among the SGAs except that olanzapine and risperidone were more effective than quetiapine or ziprasidone (Leucht et al., 2017). However, a network meta-analysis has not addressed this question.

Negative symptoms

Responses to negative symptoms often parallel effects on positive symptoms and it is often unclear whether the effects of negative symptoms may also be confounded with effects on depression or reductions in extrapyramidal side effects (EPS). Most studies have been done in patients with some negative symptoms who may also have positive and depressive symptoms. Previous meta-analyses have shown that amisulpride, clozapine, olanzapine, and risperidone are more effective than FGAs in treating negative symptoms (Leucht et al., 2009; 2017). A more recent meta-analysis on 21 double-blind studies that concentrated on studies where patients had prominent negative symptoms or patients whose symptoms were characterized as predominantly negative symptoms (i.e. with low positive or depressive symptoms) concluded that, in patients with predominant negative symptoms, amisulpride was significantly better than placebo, and olanzapine was superior to haloperidol (Krause et al., 2018). In one well-controlled study of patients with predominant negative symptoms, cariprazine was convincingly better than risperidone for reducing negative symptoms, without the confounds of its effects on positive or depressive symptoms (Nemeth et al., 2017). A recently published study with a compound in development, MIN-101(Davidson et al., 2017), which has effects on sigma-2 and 5-HT$_{2A}$ receptors, has also shown convincing effects in patients with predominant negative symptoms; this effect on negative symptoms was not mediated by changes in positive symptoms or depression.

Quality of life

Although studies for most antipsychotics show trend level or significant effects in improving quality of life and social functioning, the number of studies is too small to make any clear statements about relative efficacy of different antipsychotics.

Cognitive deficits

Cognitive impairments are believed to be core underlying deficits in schizophrenia, but there are few data to show whether particular antipsychotics are more efficacious than others for improving cognitive function. A review and meta-analysis by Guilera and associates (Guilera et al., 2009) of 18 blinded studies, 16 of which were described by their authors as double-blind, indicated small effect sizes (0.17–0.29) for SGAs in improving cognition when compared to FGAs, with significant effects on a global cognitive index, language and verbal comprehension, psychomotor function, and speed of processing. However, the data were insufficient to show whether specific SGAs were particularly more effective in improving cognitive function.

First-episode schizophrenia

In an analysis of double-blind and open studies in first-episode schizophrenia, several SGAs (amisulpride, olanzapine, ziprasidone, and risperidone) were superior in overall efficacy to haloperidol, but there was little difference between the individual SGAs, although some analyses showed olanzapine to be superior to risperidone for treating negative symptoms (Zhu et al., 2017a; 2017b).

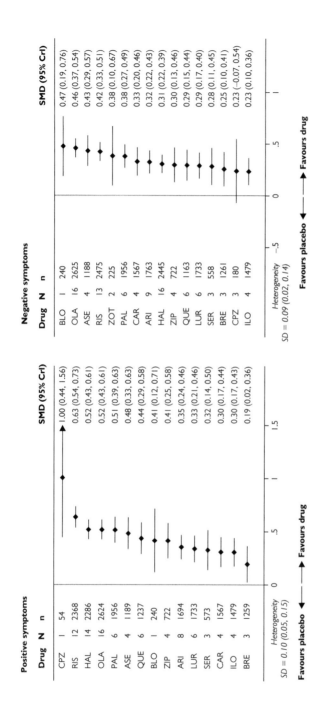

Positive symptoms

Drug	N	n	SMD (95% CrI)
CPZ	1	54	1.00 (0.44, 1.56)
RIS	12	2368	0.63 (0.54, 0.73)
HAL	14	2286	0.52 (0.43, 0.61)
OLA	16	2624	0.52 (0.43, 0.61)
PAL	6	1956	0.51 (0.39, 0.63)
ASE	4	1189	0.48 (0.33, 0.63)
QUE	6	1237	0.44 (0.29, 0.58)
BLO	1	240	0.41 (0.12, 0.71)
ZIP	4	722	0.41 (0.25, 0.58)
ARI	8	1694	0.35 (0.24, 0.46)
LUR	6	1733	0.33 (0.21, 0.46)
SER	3	573	0.32 (0.14, 0.50)
CAR	4	1567	0.30 (0.17, 0.44)
ILO	4	1479	0.30 (0.17, 0.43)
BRE	3	1259	0.19 (0.02, 0.36)

Heterogeneity
SD = 0.10 (0.05, 0.15)

Favours placebo ◄────────► Favours drug

Negative symptoms

Drug	N	n	SMD (95% CrI)
BLO	1	240	0.47 (0.19, 0.76)
OLA	16	2625	0.46 (0.37, 0.54)
ASE	4	1188	0.43 (0.29, 0.57)
RIS	13	2475	0.42 (0.33, 0.51)
ZOT	2	225	0.38 (0.10, 0.67)
PAL	6	1956	0.38 (0.27, 0.49)
CAR	4	1567	0.33 (0.20, 0.46)
ARI	9	1763	0.32 (0.22, 0.43)
HAL	16	2445	0.31 (0.22, 0.39)
ZIP	4	722	0.30 (0.13, 0.46)
QUE	6	1163	0.29 (0.15, 0.44)
LUR	6	1733	0.29 (0.17, 0.40)
SER	3	558	0.28 (0.11, 0.45)
BRE	3	1261	0.25 (0.10, 0.41)
CPZ	3	180	0.23 (−0.07, 0.54)
ILO	4	1479	0.23 (0.10, 0.36)

Heterogeneity
SD = 0.09 (0.02, 0.14)

Favours placebo ◄────────► Favours drug

Fig. 3.2 Differences in efficacy for positive and negative symptoms. Effects on positive and negative symptoms of single antipsychotics compared with placebo, pair-wise meta-analysis. These are raw effect sizes that have not been corrected for the effects of increasing placebo response over the years. The effect sizes of the single drugs have not been compared with each other. Moreover, for some drugs few data were available, making the results unreliable. For example, the results of positive symptoms for chlorpromazine are based on only one study with 54 patients. This caused uncertainty about the true effect, which is expressed by a large 95% CrI. CrI, Credible interval; SD, standard deviation; SMD, standardized mean difference. ARI, Aripiprazole; ASE, asenapine; BLO, blonanserin; BRE, brexpiprazole; CAR, cariprazine; CPZ, chlorpromazine; HAL, haloperidol; ILO, iloperidone; LUR, lurasidone; OLA, olanzapine; PAL, paliperidone; QUE, quetiapine; RIS, risperidone; SER, sertindole; ZIP, ziprasidone; ZOT, zotepine.

Reprinted from Am J Psychiatry, 174, Leucht, S., Leucht, C., Huhn, M., et al (2017). Sixty Years of Placebo-Controlled Antipsychotic Drug Trials in Acute Schizophrenia: Systematic Review, Bayesian Meta-Analysis, and Meta-Regression of Efficacy Predictors, pp 927–942, Copyright (2017), with permission from American Psychiatric Press.

Side effects of antipsychotic drugs

Antipsychotic drugs differ markedly in terms of side effects, and these differences between drugs are often greater than the efficacy differences.

Weight and diabetes

Weight gain, diabetes, and glucose and lipid abnormalities have been of particular concern with some SGAs. Large differences in weight gain are produced by different antipsychotics, with olanzapine, zotepine, clozapine, iloperidone, and chlorpromazine producing more weight gain than haloperidol, ziprasidone, lurasidone, aripiprazole, and asenapine; Fig. 3.3 (Leucht et al., 2013; 2017). However, in some studies of clozapine and olanzapine, weight gain has been positively correlated with clinical response to these antipsychotics (Ascher-Svanum et al., 2005; Czobor et al., 2002; Sharma et al., 2014). There have been few studies directly comparing diabetes risk among antipsychotics with data appropriate for inclusion in meta-analysis. The American Diabetes Association issued a consensus statement in 2004 stating that olanzapine and clozapine had the highest diabetes risk and risperidone and quetiapine had a somewhat lower risk (Asssociation and Association, 2004). An early meta-analysis using mostly retrospective studies showed a slight increase in overall diabetes risk with SGAs compared to FGAs (relative risk 1.32), but differences among specific SGAs were small (Smith et al., 2008). Two epidemiological type retrospective studies in New York state hospitals (Citrome et al., 2004) and Veterans Administration hospitals tended to show that quetiapine had the highest risk of new-onset diabetes. A cross-sectional study by Smith and associates (2005), which directly measured fasting multiple glucose-lipid levels in patients' blood, showed no significant statistical differences in any glucose- and lipid-related measures between chronic schizophrenic patients treated with clozapine, olanzapine, risperidone, or an FGA, except for an increase in triglycerides in the olanzapine- and clozapine-treated patients compared to those treated with risperidone. Several studies reported improvements in glucose and/or lipids in patients switched to aripiprazole from olanzapine, or to aripiprazole from an SGA (Spurling et al., 2007; Ganguli et al., 2011; Wani et al., 2015). A prospective Chinese study in first-episode schizophrenics comparing olanzapine, quetiapine, and aripiprazole found that olanzapine increased glucose levels, and olanzapine and quetiapine increased triglyceride levels, but no significant changes were found with aripiprazole (Zhang and Lan, 2014). Overall, there is strong evidence for certain SGAs having a greater effect on increasing weight, but definitive evidence from head-to-head comparisons concerning the relative risk of diabetes and glucose-lipid abnormalities is lacking; therefore, the differential assessment of which SGAs are associated with a significantly greater increase in diabetes risk or glucose-lipid abnormalities cannot be clearly established on the basis of current evidence.

Tolerability

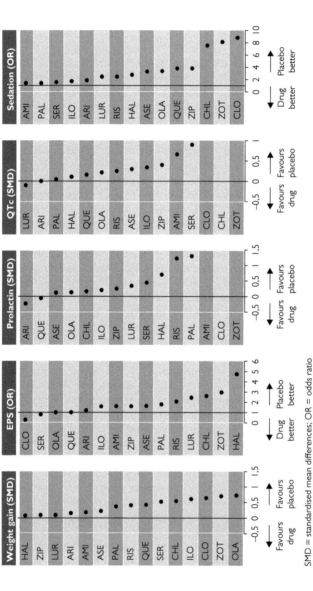

Fig. 3.3 Differences in side effects of antipsychotic drugs. Forest plots for effect sizes of antipsychotic drugs compared with placebo for side effects, network meta-analysis. Results are shown for weight gain, extrapyramidal side effects, prolactin increase, QTc prolongation, and sedation. Treatments are ranked according to their surface under the cumulative ranking (SUCRA) values. Extrapyramidal side effects are defined by at least one use of antiparkinsonian drugs. EPS, Extrapyramidal symptoms; OR, odds ratio; SMD, standardized mean difference. AMI, Amisulpride; CHL, Chlorpromazine; CLO, clozapine. Other abbreviations are defined in legend to Fig. 3.2.

SMD = standardised mean differences; OR = odds ratio

Extrapyramidal side effects and tardive dyskinesia

EPSs and movement disorders were the major side effect concerns with FGAs. Results from meta-analyses show that most SGAs are slightly to moderately superior to FGAs in reducing the frequency of EPSs, and some of the largest differences were found for clozapine and olanzapine; see Fig. 3.3 (Leucht et al., 2013; 2017). Clozapine is superior to most drugs in decreased occurrence of EPSs (usually measured in meta-analyses by lack of co-joint prescription of antiparkinsonian medications) and olanzapine is superior to zotepine, risperidone, chlorpromazine, lurasidone, ziprasidone, and haloperidol. The development of tardive dyskinesia (TD) was another major concern with FGAs. Two recent meta-analyses have shown substantially decreased rates of TD in patients treated with SGAs. A study by Carbon et al. (2017) showed a prevalence rate of TD of 30% for FGAs and 20% for SGAs, with a particularly low rate of 7.2% for patients treated with an SGA who had not been previously exposed to FGA treatment. Another study, by O'Brien in 2016, showed about a three times higher prevalence and incidence rate of TD in older patients taking FGAs rather than SGAs. TD incidence at 1 year in patients taking SGAs was 7%. However, these studies did not report results relevant to the differential effect of specific FGAs or SGAs on the development of TD, and therefore we cannot give any estimates of differential susceptibility to this side effect with different antipsychotics. In an earlier study with patients receiving FGAs, Smith and associates (Smith et al., 1978) reported that treatment with fluphenazine was the only antipsychotic with a strong positive association with TD scores.

Other side effects

Other side effects, such as prolactin elevation, QTc prolongation on electrocardiogram, and sedation may also be important, and should be taken into account when evaluating the risk–benefit ratios for choice of a specific antipsychotic. In terms of prolactin elevation, network meta-analysis showed that paliperidone, risperidone, and haloperidol had the highest prolactin increase, and aripiprazole, quetiapine, asenapine, chlorpromazine, and iloperidone did not cause more prolactin elevation than placebo (see Fig. 3.3) (Leucht et al., 2013). Although there were no placebo-controlled studies of prolactin levels with amisulpride, data from other studies show that this drug is associated with high levels of prolactin increase. Increased QTc interval can be followed in rare cases by a life-threatening ventricular tachyarrhythmia called torsade de pointes (dTDP), and this can lead to toxicity and occasional sudden death, especially in patients with much prolonged QTc at baseline or other complicating cardiac conditions. In a recent network meta-analysis (Leucht et al., 2013), sertindole, amisulpride, ziprasidone, and iloperidone were associated with the highest increase in QTc (see Fig. 3.3). Previous studies have shown that thioridazine and pimozide are also associated with increased risk of increased QTc. Sertindole has been removed from the market in some countries because of this risk, and thioridazine, an FGA, is now rarely used. Although amisulpride is associated with increased QTc and dTDP, few deaths have been reported from amisulpride overdose. Lurasidone, aripiprazole, paliperidone, and asenapine are not associated with prolonged QTc compared to placebo. In network meta-analysis, clozapine, zotepine, and chlorpromazine caused the most sedation, and amisulpride, paliperidone, sertindole, and iloperidone were not significantly more sedating than placebo.

It is important for patients with schizophrenia to maintain treatment with antipsychotic medication to reduce risk of relapse, and a measure of all-cause discontinuation of a drug may give a partial indication of acceptability to patients and doctors, which might reduce the risk of relapse. In the Clinical Antipsychotic Trials of Intervention Effectiveness (CATIE) study, olanzapine had the lowest all-cause discontinuation. In a recent network meta-analysis (Leucht et al., 2013), amisulpride, olanzapine, clozapine, paliperidone, and risperidone had significantly lower all-cause discontinuation than several other FGA or SGA drugs.

Switching to another first-line antipsychotic

If the patient has not shown an adequate response to the selected first-line antipsychotic because of lack of efficacy, or side effects that might interfere with compliance, does a switch to another antipsychotic make sense for maximizing efficacy or would increasing the dose be a better alternative?

For efficacy, first we have to consider whether the patient has been treated with an adequate dose of the first-choice antipsychotic before considering the question of switching. The analysis by Davis and Chen in 2004 provides evidence for the dose associated with 50% response (the ED_{50}) and the near maximal effective doses of many FGAs and SGAs (Table 3.2). Whilst it should be noted that tables in other articles have slightly different minimal effective doses (Leucht et al., 2014; 2016b), differences are not large. Thus Table 3.2 can be used by the treating clinician as a guide to ensure the dose of antipsychotic treatment is likely to be adequate. There is convincing evidence that high doses that significantly exceed the near maximal doses do not improve response in most patients (Davis and Chen, 2004).

The evidence base for informing a rationale choice for switching to another antipsychotic is not extensive. The appropriate design to test this includes randomization to either the same antipsychotic or the alternative antipsychotic so that the effect of duration of treatment can be controlled for. However, most studies do not use this design and consequently they cannot conclude that it was the switch to the new drug rather than increased time in treatment that was the reason for improvement in response. There is preliminary evidence that, with inadequate response to the first antipsychotic, switching to a drug with a different receptor profile may have some advantage. In a study by Kinon and associates (Kinon et al., 2010), patients treated with risperidone who did not have at least a 20% improvement on the PANSS scale by 2 weeks responded slightly but significantly better if they were switch to olanzapine rather than if they stayed

Table 3.2 The ED_{50} and near-maximal effective dose for first-generation antipsychotics (FGAs) and second-generation antipsychotics (SGAs)

Drug	ED_{50}	Near maximal effective dose
FGAs		
Chlorpromazine	150 mg/d	400–450 mg/d
Haloperidol	0.5–2 mg/d	3.5–10 mg/d
Haloperidol decanoate	25 mg/mo	100–200 mg/mo
Trifluoperazine	—	10–15 mg/d
Thiothixene	—	<10 mg/d
Fluphenazine	—	<6.9 mg/d
Fluphenazine decanoate/enantate	—	25 mg/2 wk
SGAs		
Olanzapine	9 mg/d	>16 mg/d
Olanzapine IM	>6 mg/d	>10 mg/injection
Risperidone	2 mg/d	4 mg/d
Risperidone depot	15 mg/mo	50 mg/mo
Amisulpride	50 mg/d	200 mg/d
Aripiprazole	<1.5 mg/d	10 mg/d
Quetiapine	80–215 mg/d	150–600 mg/d
Remoxipride	60 mg/d	120–240 mg/d
Sertindole	10 mg/d	12–20 mg/d
Clozapine	—	>400 mg/d
Ziprasidone, acute	63 mg/d	120–160 mg/d
Ziprasidone, maintenance	40 mg/d	80–160 mg/d

The numbers in the table are derived from dose-response curves from analysis of data from published studies or other sources of available data, where a measure of clinical response is plotted on the Y-axis vs. the log-dose plotted on the X-axis. The ED_{50} is the dose at which half the maximal clinical response is achieved. The near maximal effective doses are the doses between ED_{85} to ED_{95} on the dose response curve, which is usually at the upper plateau portion of the dose-response curve. d, day; IM, intramuscular; mo, month; wk, week.

on risperidone. In the CATIE study patients who discontinued perphenazine did better if they were switched to olanzapine or quetiapine, which have a somewhat different receptor binding profile, than if they were switched to risperidone, which has a fairly similar dopamine antagonist receptor profile. The results of a currently ongoing study, the OPTIMISE trial (Leucht et al., 2015), will provide better evidence for informing the switch strategy. This study will test the efficacy of amisulpride in first-episode schizophrenia and, if an adequate response is not shown by 4 weeks, it will test the efficacy of remaining on amisulpride versus switching to olanzapine (which has a different receptor profile); non-responders by 12 weeks will also be tested on the efficacy of switching to clozapine.

Depot versus oral antipsychotics

Several of the FGAs and SGAs are available in long-acting injectable (depot) as well as oral forms. For a patient who shows poor adherence to taking oral medication or who has frequent relapses because of stopping oral antipsychotic, depot medication might be an option. An early review by Davis and associates (1994) provided evidence for the superiority of depot versus oral antipsychotic medication for FGAs. However, a meta-analysis of randomized controlled trials with SGAs showed no advantage of depot over oral medications in preventing relapse or severe worsening of symptoms (Kishimoto et al., 2014). However, observational studies and a meta-analysis of mirror image studies (where the same patients were switched from oral to depot antipsychotics) show a clear advantage of depot versus oral medication in preventing rehospitalization and fewer hospitalization days (Kirson et al., 2013, Kishimoto et al., 2013), suggesting depots have a benefit in more naturalistic settings.

Adjunctive medication in addition to antipsychotic treatment

Will the addition of a non-antipsychotic medication help maximize clinical response in patients who have residual symptoms or less than fully adequate response?

A meta-analysis by Leucht's group (Helfer et al., 2016) provides convincing evidence that the addition of an antidepressant improves negative and depressive symptoms, with higher effect sizes seen in those patients who had either predominant or more severe negative or depressive symptoms. Importantly, there was no increase in positive symptoms with the addition of the antidepressant. Most of the reviewed studies utilized SGAs (selective serotonin reuptake inhibitors [SSRIs] or serotonin–norepinephrine reuptake inhibitors [SNRIs]) or monoamine oxidase inhibitor drugs, and some drugs or drug classes showed stronger effects, although the number of studies for each individual drug was small. Correll and associates (2017) performed a meta-analysis of previous individual meta-analyses to compare antipsychotic monotherapy to adjunctive treatment and reported that a number of add-on medications improved positive systems (with lamotrigine, and some SSRI and SNRI antidepressant type drugs and oestrogen showing the strongest effects) and for negative symptoms (with some antidepressants—SNRIs and serotonergic receptor 3 antagonists, and lamotrigine showing the strongest effects). However, in reviewing the quality of the data of the original studies on which these meta-analyses are based, they found problems in overall quality of the original studies, and a negative correlation between ratings of quality of the underlying individual studies and the effect size of the difference between add-on therapy from placebo. Therefore, they concluded that many of the statistically significant positive effects of add-on treatments may have a relatively low or confounded evidence level.

Recommendations for maximizing first-line antipsychotic response

Choice of first-line antipsychotic

How might the comparative data on efficacy and side effects be used by clinicians and patients to choose the most appropriate antipsychotic for treatment of acute symptom episodes in patients with first episode or relapsing schizophrenia?

Many of the SGAs are now off patent, and others will be coming off patent in the next few years, so differential cost is a less important consideration than it was in the 1990s and early 2000s. Because almost all of the SGAs have a reduced risk of EPS and TD than the FGAs and many are now available both in oral and long-acting intramuscular form, treatment with an SGA should be a first choice in most cases. The choice among SGAs should consider the patient's personal history in response to antipsychotics in the past and the risk–benefit consideration of efficacy for overall or specific symptoms versus side effects. As clozapine has shown strong efficacy and relatively low incidence of standard side effects, except for increased sedation and the low risk of agranulocytosis, it might be considered a good first-line treatment that has been underutilized. However, most of the data for clozapine are based on older studies against placebo, and most of the other data for clozapine are in treatment-resistant patients who are non-responders to traditional antipsychotic medications. Results of ongoing studies in Europe using clozapine as a first-line treatment in non-treatment-resistant patients with schizophrenia may provide information to better inform psychiatrists on the standard use of clozapine as a first-line treatment. Outside of clozapine, olanzapine and amisulpride have high acceptability and relatively higher efficacy for both positive and negative symptoms. In patients where weight gain or diabetes is not a stronger concern than efficacy, olanzapine would have a favourable benefit–risk ratio and might be given higher consideration. In cases where there are no serious cardiac risks and increased prolactin is not considered of primary importance, amisulpride should be given stronger consideration. However, this drug is only available in certain countries and not in the United States. Where avoiding weight gain and glucose-lipid abnormalities are prime considerations, and the development of an akathisia anxiety-like side effect is not worrisome, aripiprazole should be given stronger consideration. Risperidone has a good efficacy profile but would likely cause more prolactin elevation, sedation and EPSs than other SGAs, especially at higher doses. When the focus is on treating negative symptoms of schizophrenia, amisulpride or olanzapine might be given special consideration, as well as clozapine. Also, a more recently approved antipsychotic, cariprazine, has convincing evidence from one study showing it had strong effects on negative symptoms. However, this drug is likely to be more expensive because it will be on patent protection for many years, and the positive results of this single study need to be replicated and compared with drugs other than risperidone. If confirmed by further studies and approved by oversight agencies in different countries, a new drug currently in development, MIN-101, might also be given higher consideration for treatment of negative symptoms, but may be primarily used as an add-on treatment if control of positive symptoms is also important. The current literature does not provide strong evidence for choosing among the SGAs for treatment of first-episode schizophrenia specifically, although a few of the SGAs are more efficacious than haloperidol.

Switching to another antipsychotic

Before considering a switch to another antipsychotic if there is inadequate response after 2–4 weeks of treatment with an adequate dose, the clinician should evaluate whether the patient has been treated with an adequate dose of the chosen first-line antipsychotic. Since occasional patients may be fast metabolizers and have very low blood levels even on adequate dosing, it may be prudent to check a drug blood level. Although there is not an extensive evidence base for choosing a drug to switch to, a choice of another antipsychotic with a different receptor profile (such as a switch from amisulpride to olanzapine) may be the most reasonable, with a strategy of cross-tapering the original antipsychotic and new drug over 1–2 weeks. If a patient shows poor compliance, especially with frequent relapses, switching from an oral to depot form of the same first-line antipsychotic which showed an adequate response would help to maximize long-term response.

Adjunctive medication treatment

If depression or negative symptoms are prominent in the symptom picture, the addition of an SSRI or SNRI may be worth a trial. For depressive symptoms, there is an evidence base to support the use of duloxetine, trazodone, or sertraline, and for negative symptoms duloxetine, mirtazapine, and several of the SSRIs would be evidence-based choices.

In making the choice for first-line antipsychotic treatment or switches and adjunctive treatment, it is clinically important for the treating psychiatrist to report response and side effects clearly in an easily understandable manner so that future psychiatrists can evaluate prior treatment responses and treatment side effects. The development of a template for standard reporting may be helpful.

Conclusions

Our review of recent studies using meta-analysis techniques has provided evidence that all antipsychotics are not equal in efficacy or in the severity of different side effects. Comparative analysis and rankings from network meta-analyses can provide guidance to clinicians in choosing the most appropriate antipsychotic for first-line treatment, if used in conjunction with available information of the patient's history of previous clinical response or higher risks for specific side effects. More evidence is needed to assess the best alternative antipsychotic to switch to if there is not an adequate response to the first choice after 2–4 weeks of treatment with an adequate dose. More evidence is also needed to establish how much clozapine should be supported as a first-line treatment for patients who are *not* classified as antipsychotic-resistant or chronic non-responders. Ongoing studies may begin to provide more evidence to inform better responses to these two questions in the next few years.

REFERENCES

Ascher-Svanum, H., Stensland, M. D., Kinon, B. J., Tollefson, G. D. (2005). Weight gain as a prognostic indicator of therapeutic improvement during acute treatment of schizophrenia with placebo or active antipsychotic. *J Psychopharmacol*, 19, 110–17.

Association, A. D., Association, A. P. (2004). Consensus development conference on antipsychotic drugs and obesity and diabetes. *Diabetes Care*, 27, 596–601.

Borenstein, M., Hedges, L., Higgins, J., Rothstein, H. (2009). *Introduction to Meta-Analysis*. West Sussex: John Wiley and Sons.

Carbon, M., Hsieh, C. H., Kane, J. M., Correll, C. U. (2017). Tardive dyskinesia prevalence in the period of second-generation antipsychotic use: a meta-analysis. *J Clin Psychiatry*, 78, e264–e278.

Citrome, L., Jaffe, A., Levine, J., Allingham, B., Robinson, J. (2004). Relationship between antipsychotic medication treatment and new cases of diabetes among psychiatric inpatients. *Psychiatr Serv*, 55, 1006–13.

Correll, C. U., Rubio, J. M., Inczedy-Farkas, G., Birnbaum, M. L., Kane, J. M., Leucht, S. (2017). Efficacy of 42 pharmacologic cotreatment strategies added to antipsychotic monotherapy in schizophrenia: systematic overview and quality appraisal of the meta-analytic evidence. *JAMA Psychiatry*, 74, 675–84.

Czobor, P., Volavka, J., Sheitman, B., et al. (2002). Antipsychotic-induced weight gain and therapeutic response: a differential association. *J Clin Psychopharmacol*, 22, 244–51.

Davidson, M., Saoud, J., Staner, C., et al. (2017). Efficacy and safety of MIN-101: a 12-week randomized, double-blind, placebo-controlled trial of a new drug in development for the treatment of negative symptoms in schizophrenia. *Am J Psychiatry*, 174, 1195–202.

Davis, J. M., Chen, N. (2004). Dose response and dose equivalence of antipsychotics. *J Clin Psychopharmacol*, 24, 192–208.

Davis, J. M., Matalon, L., Watanabe, M. D., Blake, L., Metalon, L. (1994). Depot antipsychotic drugs. Place in therapy. *Drugs*, 47, 741–73.

Ganguli, R., Brar, J. S., Garbut, R., Chang, C. C., Basu, R. (2011). Changes in weight and other metabolic indicators in persons with schizophrenia following a switch to aripiprazole. *Clin Schizophr Relat Psychoses*, 5, 75–9.

Guilera, G., Pino, O., Gomex-Benito, J., Rojo, J. (2009). Antipsychotic effects on cognition in schizophrenia: a meta-analysis of randomized controlled trials. *Eur J Psychatr*, 23, 77–89.

Guttmacher, M. S. (1964). Phenothiazine treatment in acute schizophrenia; effectiveness: The National Institute of Mental Health Psychopharmacology Service Center Collaborative Study Group. *Arch Gen Psychiatry*, 10, 246–61.

Helfer, B., Samara, M. T., Huhn, M., et al. (2016). Efficacy and safety of antidepressants added to antipsychotics for schizophrenia: a systematic review and meta-analysis. *Am J Psychiatry*, 173, 876–86.

Higgins, J., Green, S. (2008). *Cochrane Handbook for Systematic Review of Interventions*. West Sussex: John Wiley and Sons.

Kinon, B. J., Chen, L., Ascher-Svanum, H., et al. (2010). Early response to antipsychotic drug therapy as a clinical marker of subsequent response in the treatment of schizophrenia. *Neuropsychopharmacology*, 35, 581–90.

Kirson, N. Y., Weiden, P. J., Yermakov, S., et al. (2013). Efficacy and effectiveness of depot versus oral antipsychotics in schizophrenia: synthesizing results across different research designs. *J Clin Psychiatry*, 74, 568–75.

Kishimoto, T., Nitta, M., Borenstein, M., Kane, J. M., Correll, C. U. (2013). Long-acting injectable versus oral antipsychotics in schizophrenia: a systematic review and meta-analysis of mirror-image studies. *J Clin Psychiatry*, 74, 957–65.

Kishimoto, T., Robenzadeh, A., Leucht, C., et al. (2014). Long-acting injectable vs oral antipsychotics for relapse prevention in schizophrenia: a meta-analysis of randomized trials. *Schizophr Bull*, 40, 192–213.

Krause, M., Zhu, Y., Huhn, M., et al. (2018). Antipsychotic drugs for patients with schizophrenia and predominant or prominent negative symptoms: a systematic review and meta-analysis. *Eur Arch Psychiatry Clin Neurosci*, doi: 10.1007/s00406-018-0869-3.

Leucht, S., Corves, C., Arbter, D., Engel, R. R., Li, C., Davis, J. M. (2009). Second-generation versus first-generation antipsychotic drugs for schizophrenia: a meta-analysis. *Lancet*, 373, 31–41.

Leucht, S., Cipriani, A., Spineli, L., et al. (2013). Comparative efficacy and tolerability of 15 antipsychotic drugs in schizophrenia: a multiple-treatments meta-analysis. *Lancet*, 382(9896), 951–62.

Leucht, S., Samara, M., Heres, S., Patel, M. X., Woods, S. W., Davis, J. M. (2014). Dose equivalents for second-generation antipsychotics: the minimum effective dose method. *Schizophr Bull*, 40, 314–26.

CHAPTER 3

Leucht, S., Winter-Van Rossum, I., Heres, S., et al. (2015). The optimization of treatment and management of schizophrenia in Europe (OPTiMiSE) trial: rationale for its methodology and a review of the effectiveness of switching antipsychotics. *Schizophr Bull*, 41, 549–58.

Leucht, S., Chaimani, A., Cipriani, A. S., Davis, J. M., Furukawa, T. A., Salanti, G. (2016a). Network meta-analyses should be the highest level of evidence in treatment guidelines. *Eur Arch Psychiatry Clin Neurosci*, 266, 477–80.

Leucht, S., Samara, M., Heres, S., Davis, J. M. (2016b). Dose equivalents for antipsychotic drugs: the DDD method. *Schizophr Bull*, 42 (Suppl. 1), S90–4.

Leucht, S., Leucht, C., Huhn, M., et al. (2017). Sixty years of placebo-controlled antipsychotic drug trials in acute schizophrenia: systematic review, Bayesian meta-analysis, and meta-regression of efficacy predictors. *Am J Psychiatry*, 174, 927–42.

Lieberman, J., Stroup, T., McEvoy, J., et al. and Clinical Antipsychotic Trials of Intervention Effectiveness (CATIE) Investigators. (2005). Effectiveness of antipsychotic drugs in patients with chronic schizophrenia. *N Engl J Med*, 353, 1209–23.

Nemeth, G., Laszlovszky, I., Czobor, P., et al. (2017). Cariprazine versus risperidone monotherapy for treatment of predominant negative symptoms in patients with schizophrenia: a randomised, double-blind, controlled trial. *Lancet*, 389, 1103–13.

O'Brien, A. (2016). Comparing the risk of tardive dyskinesia in older adults with first-generation and second-generation antipsychotics: a systematic review and meta-analysis. *Int J Geriatr Psychiatry*, 31, 683–93.

Sharma, E., Rao, N. P., Venkatasubramanian, G. (2014). Association between antipsychotic-induced metabolic side-effects and clinical improvement: a review on the evidence for 'metabolic threshold'. *Asian J Psychiatr*, 8, 12–21.

Smith, M., Hopkins, D., Peveler, R. C., Holt, R. I., Woodward, M., Ismail, K. (2008). First- v. second-generation antipsychotics and risk for diabetes in schizophrenia: systematic review and meta-analysis. *Br J Psychiatry*, 192, 406–11.

Smith, R., Lindenmayer, J.-P., Bark, N., Warner-Cohen, J., Vaidhyanathaswamy, S., Khandat, A. (2005). Clozapine, risperidone, olanzapine, and conventional antipsychotic drug effects on glucose, lipids, and leptin in schizophrenic patients. *Int J Neuropsychopharmacology*, 8, 183–94.

Smith, R. C., Strizich, M., Klass, D. (1978). Drug history and tardive dyskinesia. *Am J Psychiatry*, 135, 1402–3.

Spurling, R. D., Lamberti, J. S., Olsen, D., Tu, X., Tang, W. (2007). Changes in metabolic parameters with switching to aripiprazole from another second-generation antipsychotic: a retrospective chart review. *J Clin Psychiatry*, 68, 406–9.

Wani, R. A., Dar, M. A., Chandel, R. K., et al. (2015). Effects of switching from olanzapine to aripiprazole on the metabolic profiles of patients with schizophrenia and metabolic syndrome: a double-blind, randomized, open-label study. *Neuropsychiatr Dis Treat*, 11, 685–93.

Zhang, S., Lan, G. (2014). Prospective 8-week trial on the effect of olanzapine, quetiapine, and aripiprazole on blood glucose and lipids among individuals with first-onset schizophrenia. *Shanghai Arch Psychiatry*, 26, 339–46.

Zhu, Y., Krause, M., Huhn, M., et al. (2017a). Antipsychotic drugs for the acute treatment of patients with a first episode of schizophrenia: a systematic review with pairwise and network meta-analyses. *Lancet Psychiatry, 4,* 694–705.

Zhu, Y., Li, C., Huhn, M., et al. (2017b). How well do patients with a first episode of schizophrenia respond to antipsychotics: a systematic review and meta-analysis. *Eur Neuropsychopharmacol, 27,* 835–44.

CHAPTER 4

Epidemiology, impact, and predictors of treatment-resistant schizophrenia

John Lally and James H. MacCabe

KEY POINTS

- Treatment-resistant schizophrenia (TRS) is a disabling psychotic disorder that affects approximately 30% of those diagnosed with schizophrenia.

- In a significant proportion of patients, illness is treatment-resistant from the first presentation (primary TRS), whilst in a smaller proportion (about 20%) treatment resistance develops during the course of treating the illness.

- TRS is associated with reduced quality of life, increased hospital use, and greater social and economic burden, all of which are more affected than in schizophrenia in general.

- A number of sociodemographic, clinical, and biological risk factors may be useful in identifying patients who have a treatment-resistant illness, although further work is required to develop a diagnostic test that can be used in routine clinical practice.

Treatment-resistant schizophrenia

Approximately 50–70% of patients with a first episode of schizophrenia (FES) will respond to antipsychotic medication, with this response rate falling to 20% for those who require a second trial (Agid et al., 2011). Although antipsychotics are the mainstay of treatment for schizophrenia, as many as one in three individuals do not respond to non-clozapine antipsychotics and are described as having 'treatment-resistant schizophrenia' (TRS).

Defining treatment resistance

Previously, a lack of consensus on TRS criteria led to variation in prevalence rates, reflecting the use of narrower (Kane et al., 1988) versus broader definitions (Conley and Kelly, 2001; NICE, 2014). In the UK, TRS is defined as non-response to two sequential trials of antipsychotic medication of adequate dose and duration (NICE, 2014), at which point the antipsychotic clozapine is indicated.

International consensus guidelines on defining treatment resistance (and response) in schizophrenia have recently been developed (see Chapter 2) (Howes et al., 2017). According to these guidelines, three key elements define the concept of TRS: 1) a confirmed diagnosis of schizophrenia; 2) pharmacological treatment of adequate duration (6–8 weeks), dose, and compliance; and 3) persistence of significant symptoms despite adequate treatment.

An important consideration when assessing treatment resistance in schizophrenia is to differentiate between actual treatment resistance and pseudoresistance, which may be attributable to non-adherence, inadequate treatment duration or dose, or inadequate treatment owing to suboptimal plasma antipsychotic concentrations (McCutcheon et al., 2018; Lally and MacCabe, 2015). In some studies, treatment intolerance may be mistaken for treatment resistance, as it is not always possible to determine the reasoning underlying a change in antipsychotic, especially when using retrospective data.

Recovery and outcome in schizophrenia

Antipsychotic treatment failure and intolerability comes with a high clinical and economic cost. A systematic review and meta-analysis of remission and recovery in first-episode psychosis (FEP) in 5000 people with FES found a recovery rate of 30% (95% confidence interval [CI] 19.7–43.6, $n = 12$ studies) at 5-year follow-up, with 56.0% (95% CI 47.5–64.1, $n = 25$ studies) meeting criteria for symptomatic remission at 7.5-year follow-up (Lally et al., 2017). This study highlighted a better long-term prognosis in FES, and a more positive outlook for people diagnosed with schizophrenia than had been previously suggested (Jaaskelainen et al., 2013). Estimates of the prevalence of TRS derived from clinical samples should be interpreted with this in mind; the prevalence of TRS is likely to be overestimated in most studies, as patients with good outcomes tend not to be included because they are discharged from services.

Prevalence of treatment-resistant schizophrenia

Cohort studies have identified a consistent rate of approximately 20–30% of those with schizophrenia meeting criteria for treatment resistance (Lally et al., 2016a; Wimberley et al., 2016b; Demjaha et al., 2017). In a recent Danish nationwide register study with a follow-up of up to 15 years (median follow-up 9 years), the prevalence rate of TRS was 21% (TRS criteria defined by clozapine initiation or hospital admission after at least two different periods of antipsychotic monotherapy) (Wimberley et al., 2016b). A prospective study of risk factors for TRS in FES identified a prevalence rate of 34% for TRS over a 5-year follow-up (Lally et al., 2016a). A longitudinal study of 244 patients with FES identified that approximately 20% of patients failed to show a response to sequential trials of olanzapine and risperidone, with 75% (21/28) responding to a third trial of clozapine (Agid et al., 2011).

The highest rate of TRS (60%) was identified in a cohort of inpatients with a history of hospitalization for at least 24 months in the past 5 years. This estimate was based on a cohort of exclusively long-term hospitalized patients, introducing a sampling bias enriching the sample for treatment-resistant patients and an overestimate of the prevalence (Essock et al., 1996b). The increased prevalence of treatment resistance in those most debilitated and requiring intensive support was replicated in the UK, when a prevalence rate of 50% was identified in 150 assertive outreach and former rehabilitation inpatients, a hospital-monitored group who are known to be difficult to treat (Mortimer et al., 2010).

A retrospective analysis of schizophrenia patients in New York state identified prevalence rates for TRS of 58% in inpatients and 24% in outpatients (Terkelsen and Grosser, 1990). A French study identified a prevalence rate of 5% (the lowest in the literature), and was likely an underestimate based on restrictive inclusion criteria, including persistence of illness for at least 3 years and inpatient status (Vanelle, 1995). According to a narrow definition of TRS adopted (persisting psychotic symptoms from illness onset or persisting symptoms subsequent to relapses), treatment resistance was observed in 15–30% of patients in a longitudinal cohort study of 15 years, with 10% of patients not responding to any treatment (Wiersma et al., 1998). The variation in prevalence rate based on TRS criteria is illustrated in a random, stratified group of schizophrenia patients ($n = 293$) treated by a county mental health system in 1991 (Juarez-Reyes et al., 1995), in which a TRS prevalence of 42.9% was identified when using the Food and Drug Administration (FDA) criteria for using clozapine compared to a prevalence of 12.9% when applying the more conservative criteria of Kane et al. (this lower rate was exacerbated by the low number of patients who had three failed antipsychotic trials documented) (Kane et al., 1988).

While there are outliers, given the variations in definition and the biases, most estimates of the prevalence of TRS in schizophrenia seem to converge at 20–30%. Given the worldwide lifetime prevalence of schizophrenia of 0.5–0.7% (McGrath et al., 2008; Simeone et al., 2015), the lifetime prevalence of TRS can be estimated at approximately 0.2% in the adult population (Bachmann et al., 2017). Worldwide, approximately 38.2 million people have a diagnosis of schizophrenia. A conservative estimate is that 20% of those (i.e. 7.6 million) will meet the criteria for TRS.

Economic costs of schizophrenia and treatment-resistant schizophrenia

The cost of care for individuals with schizophrenia is very high, with direct costs in western countries ranging between 1.6% and 2.6% of total healthcare expenditures (Davies and Drummond, 1994). Moreover, schizophrenia is the eighth leading cause of disability-adjusted life years (DALYs) worldwide in the age group 15–44 years (WHO, 2001). The cost of care was estimated to be £6.7 billion in the UK alone in 2004/05 (Mangalore and Knapp, 2007), and the total societal cost in England in 2007 was estimated at £11.8 billion per year, with a cost to the public sector of £7.2 billion (Andrew et al., 2012). In the USA, direct medical costs associated with TRS are conservatively estimated at over $34 billion (Kennedy et al., 2014). It has been estimated that hospitalization costs and total health resource utilizations for TRS are 10-fold higher than those for non-TRS and that up to 80% of the total yearly health costs associated with schizophrenia in the USA are attributed to TRS (Kennedy et al., 2014). TRS hospitalization costs and total health resource utilizations were 60- and 19-fold higher, respectively, than for the general US population (Kennedy et al., 2014). In the UK, the 10% of patients with schizophrenia who have a long-term disabling course, many of whom have TRS illnesses, account for 80% of the total lifetime direct costs for schizophrenia (Andrew et al., 2012).

Hospitalization costs are the main component of the higher total healthcare costs associated with TRS (Knapp, 2004), with approximately half of these costs attributable to hospital admissions (Kennedy et al., 2014). Health economic evidence suggests that the use of clozapine has the potential to improve the use of health and social service resources in TRS (Aitchison and Kerwin, 1997), as the use of clozapine is associated with shorter inpatient admissions (Kirwan et al., 2017; Hayhurst et al., 2002), lower rates of relapse, and reduced rehospitalization (Taipale et al., 2017; Stroup et al., 2016; Essock et al., 1996a; Land et al., 2017). A cost–benefit model study within the Veterans Health Administration (VHA) in the USA, comparing costs and monetizing benefits associated with clozapine use and non-use in TRS, identified that, if 20% of TRS cases started clozapine, this would be associated with an average annual reduction in health costs of $22,444 per patient treated with clozapine, and if there were to be a doubling in clozapine rates of use, a total direct healthcare cost saving of $80 million per annum would be made (based on an estimated VHA population of 18,000 TRS patients) (Goren et al., 2016).

The economic impact of TRS extends beyond health expenditure costs. Patients with TRS have more functional impairment in the community setting than patients with treatment-refractory bipolar affective disorder, depression, and anxiety disorders (Iasevoli et al., 2016). The mean quality of life of a person with TRS is estimated to be 20% lower than that of a person with treatment-responsive schizophrenia (Kennedy et al., 2014).

There are limited data on lost productivity due to TRS, with no reliable data on employment rates in TRS available to date. It has been estimated that unemployment in TRS exceeds 70% (Kennedy et al., 2014), but this is likely to be an underestimate. An average employment rate of 21.5% was identified for people with schizophrenia living in France, Germany, and the UK ($n = 1208$), although, for those with a continuous course of illness (and likely a high proportion meeting the criteria for TRS), that rate fell to 8.2% (Marwaha et al., 2007). An Israeli nationwide survey of hospitalized patients with severe mental illness identified that 10.6% of people with a diagnosis of schizophrenia and a single lifetime hospital admission earned minimum wage or above, compared to 5.8% of those with schizophrenia and multiple hospital admissions (a proxy for a more severe illness course and TRS) (Davidson et al., 2016).

People with TRS have increased rates of alcohol abuse (51%) and substance abuse (51%), compared to those with non-TRS (27–35% alcohol abuse and 28–35% substance abuse), with suicidal ideation in 44% of those with TRS (Kennedy et al., 2014). The lifetime suicide risk in TRS and non-TRS is thought to be equivalent, equating to a 5% lifetime risk; this is a major contributor to premature mortality in this patient group (Palmer et al., 2005).

Although TRS has high social and economic costs, early identification of patients who might benefit from clozapine or alternative treatments has the potential to improve clinical outcomes and minimize the social and functional disability that results from prolonged psychosis (Lewis et al., 2006; Wheeler et al., 2009; Stroup et al., 2016).

Risk factors for treatment resistance

Despite affecting around one-third of people with schizophrenia, risk factors predictive for TRS have not been investigated widely. Further, while there is a large literature investigating predictors of treatment response and remission from illness onset (Carbon and Correll, 2014; Menezes et al., 2006), treatment resistance has only recently been examined longitudinally as an outcome measure in FEP (Lally et al., 2016a; Demjaha et al., 2017).

Prediction of TRS needs to be viewed in relation to potential premorbid risk factors but also to the stage of illness and to the temporal relationship between the onset of schizophrenia and the emergence of TRS.

Although a few potential risk factors for treatment resistance, such as poor premorbid functioning, living in less urban areas, comorbid personality disorder, longer duration of untreated psychosis, greater severity of negative symptoms, and a younger age of illness onset have been suggested (Schennach et al., 2012; Ortiz et al., 2013; Vanelle et al., 1994; Meltzer, 1997; Frank et al., 2015; Wimberley et al., 2016b; Martin and Mowry, 2016; Lally et al., 2016a; Demjaha et al., 2017), the predictive value of specific clinical and demographic factors on treatment resistance in FES has not yet been widely investigated (Lin et al., 2008).

Early age of onset and male sex are the most consistent predictors for the development of TRS (Lally et al., 2016a). This is supported by earlier findings that those with TRS were more likely to be male and have an average 2-year earlier age of illness onset (mean 19.4 years, standard deviation [SD] 4.7) compared to non-TRS patients (mean 21.2 years, SD 6.1) (Meltzer et al., 1997), and younger age of illness onset (although not male gender) was replicated in a nationwide longitudinal cohort study of risk factors for TRS (Wimberley et al., 2016b).

This Danish nationwide registry study using a treatment-based proxy for TRS identified a number of patient-related factors, including younger age and rural living, and disease-related factors, including a higher number of hospitalizations, inpatient admission at first contact, and prior medication use before diagnosis of FES (including antipsychotic use, antidepressant use, and benzodiazepine use), a history of suicide attempt and additional psychiatric diagnoses (in addition to schizophrenia) being predictive for the development of treatment resistance (Wimberley et al., 2016b). A higher level of functional impairment, categorized as a Global Assessment of Functioning score <30, was associated with an increased risk of treatment resistance within 2 years of first diagnosis with schizophrenia (Horsdal et al., 2017).

In contrast to urban living being a recognized risk factor for general schizophrenia, an inverse association between TRS and urbanicity has been identified (Wimberley et al., 2016a), with the hypothesis that TRS, being a non-dopaminergic subtype of schizophrenia, is not driven by increased dopamine synthesis mediated by increased stress and urban living.

Neurochemical imaging markers

There have been putative central and peripheral biomarkers identified in schizophrenia. In addition, numerous studies have identified peripheral circulatory, inflammatory, and immunological abnormalities in schizophrenia patients, with evidence that some cytokines, such as interleukins (IL)-1β and -6, transforming growth factor (TGF)-β, and IL-12, may be possible state markers in TRS, while interferon (INF)-γ, tumour necrosis factor (TNF)-α, and IL-2R may be possible trait markers in TRS (Miller et al., 2011).

Neuroimaging techniques have been utilized to demonstrate that those who show a poor response to antipsychotic treatment in FEP have higher levels of glutamate in the anterior cingulate cortex than patients who respond well. Further, high glutamate levels are associated with increased levels of negative symptomatology and poor levels of functioning (Egerton et al., 2012). Neuroimaging studies have provided evidence that there are biological differences between treatment-resistant and treatment-responsive schizophrenia: TRS patients demonstrated higher glutamate levels in the anterior cingulate cortex (Demjaha et al., 2014), with relatively normal dopamine functioning, in comparison to treatment-responsive patients (Demjaha et al., 2012). The potential role of glutamate in the pathogenesis of general schizophrenia is supported by recent findings from the Psychiatric Genomics Consortium and other studies, in which genome-wide significant associations with schizophrenia have been observed in glutamate system genes, such as GRM3, GRIN2A, GRIA1, and GRIN2B (Schizophrenia Working Group of the Psychiatric Genomics Consortium, 2014; Kirov et al., 2012). In TRS, a handful of studies have investigated glutamate system genes in relation to clozapine response. These have largely focused on variants in GRIN2B, which codes for the 2B subunit of the N-methyl-D-aspartate (NMDA) receptor, although with results that have been largely negative to date (Taylor et al., 2016).

Genetic markers

Pharmacogenomic studies of TRS risk and clozapine response and tolerability have produced conflicting results secondary to heterogeneous inclusion criteria and other patient characteristics that act as confounding factors (Lally et al., 2016b). Genetic association studies in TRS have identified some associations between TRS and candidate genes, though with little or no replicability. The catechol-ortho-methyltransferase (COMT) L/L genotype was more common in those with TRS compared to non-TRS patients (Inada et al., 2003). Brain-derived neurotrophic factor (BDNF) gene polymorphisms (s11030104 (odds ratio [OR] 2.57), rs10501087 (OR 2.19), and rs6265 (Val66Met)) (OR 2.08) were associated with treatment resistance in Caucasian patients (Zhang et al., 2013), but the Val66Met polymorphism was not found in an earlier study (Anttila et al., 2005). Mixed results in serotonin receptor (5HTR2A, 5HTR3A, 5HTR4) candidate gene studies have been found, with the 5HT2RA C/C genotype found in treatment resistance (Anttila et al., 2007; Joober et al., 1999), but this was not replicated in later candidate gene studies (Ji et al., 2008). A systematic review identified nine gene association studies comparing patients with TRS and treatment-responsive schizophrenia, with some of the individual study findings being suggestive of gene associations with TRS, although none of these survived adjustment for multiple comparisons (Gillespie et al., 2017). Table 4.1 summarizes findings from candidate gene studies in TRS.

Table 4.1 Candidate gene studies in treatment-resistant schizophrenia

Gene	Variant	Reported association
Dopamine		
DRD3	Bal I polymorphism	Decreased homozygosity in TR (Krebs et al., 1998)
Catechol-ortho-methyltransferase (COMT)	COMT gene	L/L genotype more common in TRS compared to non-TRS patients (Inada et al., 2003)
Serotonin		
5-HTR2A	T102C	C/C genotype in treatment resistance (Joober et al., 1999) C/C genotype TR (females only) (Anttila et al., 2007)
5-HTR3A	5-HT2RA polymorphism rs6313	No significant association observed between TRS and 5-HTR2A,
5-HTR4	5-HTR3A polymorphisms rs1062613 and rs1176713 5-HTR4 polymorphisms rs2278392 and rs3734119	5-HTR3A, and 5-HTR4 alleles (Ji et al., 2008)

continued >

Table 4.1 Candidate gene studies in treatment-resistant schizophrenia (*continued*)

Gene	Variant	Reported association
Brain- derived neurotrophic factor (BDNF) gene	BDNF gene polymorphisms rs11030104 (OR 2.57), rs10501087 (OR 2.19) and rs6265 (Val66Met)) Val66Met (G169A) polymorphism rs6265 C270T polymorphism BDNF dinucleotide repeat (168 bp) polymorphism	Increased frequency in treatment-resistant patients (defined by clozapine use) compared to non-clozapine-treated patients (Zhang et al., 2013). No difference between treatment-resistant and treatment-responsive patients (Anttila et al., 2005). Increased short allele (168 bp) of the BDNF dinucleotide repeat polymorphism in treatment-resistant compared to treatment-responsive patients (Krebs et al., 2000)
Tryptophan hydroxylase (TPH) enzyme gene	TPH1 gene	TPH1 A779C C/A genotype C/A genotype increased in treatment resistance (Anttila et al., 2007)
Guanine nucleotide binding protein gene	G-protein beta-3 subunit (*GNB3*) gene	No difference in frequency of C825T C/T alleles between treatment-resistant and treatment-responsive patients (Anttila et al., 2007)
Reelin gene	5'UTR (CCG repeat) polymorphism	CCG10 reelin alleles increased in treatment resistance (Goldberger et al., 2005)
Regulator of g-protein signalling (*RGS4*) gene	*RGS4* gene	No difference in frequency of *RGS4* (T > G, Rs 951436) between treatment-resistant and treatment-responsive patients
Human leukocyte antigen (HLA) genotypes	HLA-A1 allele	HLA-A1 allele increased in treatment resistance (Lahdelma et al., 1998). No increased frequency of HLA-A1 allele in treatment-resistant compared to treatment-responsive patients (Meged et al., 1999)

This table summarizes the candidate gene studies that have investigated associations with treatment-resistant schizophrenia (TRS) compared to treatment-responsive schizophrenia. Bp, Base pairs; OR, odds ratio.

In summary, the use of pharmacogenomic testing to identify TRS and patients who may respond to clozapine remains a long way off, and the ability of clinicians to use existing pharmacogenomic findings to predict TRS and personalize clozapine treatment and identify patients at high risk of treatment failure or adverse events is not an immediately realistic possibility.

Two distinct types of treatment resistance

Recently, we reported a 5-year prospective study of 246 patients with FES, of whom 34% were classified as treatment-resistant over the course of follow-up. In this, the first prospective study to examine the course of treatment resistance after FES, 70% (n = 56) of treatment-resistant patients and 23% of the total study population (n = 246) were treatment-resistant from illness onset. Our findings indicate that two distinct patterns of treatment resistance develop in patients, with the majority displaying treatment resistance from the onset (early treatment resistance (E-TR), within 6 months of first onset of schizophrenia with no period of remission from illness onset) and a smaller subset of patients developing treatment resistance after periods of relapse (late treatment resistance (L-TR), with an initial antipsychotic response and symptomatic remission for at least 6 months' duration, with a later non-response to the ongoing use of non-clozapine antipsychotics, meeting the criteria for treatment resistance) (Lally et al., 2016a).

The finding that 23% of the total population met the criteria for treatment resistance from illness onset indicates that this course of illness is not associated with prior antipsychotic use and raises the possibility that it may be a distinctive and homogeneous schizophrenia subgroup, in line with evidence that there are biological differences between treatment-resistant and treatment-responsive schizophrenia (Demjaha et al., 2012; 2014). This finding mirrors the rate of 20% who displayed 'chronicity' from illness outset in an FEP population (Wiersma et al., 1998), although it is higher than a previous finding of 10% of FEP cases with no response to antipsychotics at the end of the first year of treatment (Robinson et al., 1999). Further, our finding that 70% of the treatment-resistant group displayed E-TR is similar to an earlier study in established schizophrenia, which identified that over half of patients with 'poor outcomes' remained psychotic from illness onset (Kolakowska et al., 1985). The high rates of early resistance of those with treatment resistance in this population is an important finding, which needs to be viewed in relation to the delay in clozapine use which exists in clinical practice (Howes et al., 2012), specifically the underuse of clozapine within the first 1–2 years of illness presentation.

A minority of those with treatment resistance (i.e. 30%) initially responded to antipsychotic medications before developing L-TR (Lally et al., 2016a). One possibility is that the loss of antipsychotic response may be because of the emergence of dopamine receptor supersensitivity in these cases. Dopamine supersensitivity is postulated to occur due to upregulation of dopamine receptors and neural adaptation (Iyo et al., 2013; Chouinard, 1991), and it has been estimated that 50% of treatment resistance might be because of the emergence of dopamine supersensitivity (Chouinard and Chouinard, 2008). Conversely, previous studies have found that over the course of illness, approximately one in six develops a lack of antipsychotic response subsequent to relapses (Wiersma et al., 1998; Emsley et al., 2012), a lower rate of L-TR than the 30% identified in our study. It may be that there was a greater delay in treatment change for patients who relapsed in our naturalistic clinical setting than in the closely monitored setting of the open label study of Emsley et al. (2012), in which patients had a treatment initiation at the time of relapse. This delay in antipsychotic use may have contributed to the higher rate of L-TR that we have identified, suggesting that relapses themselves may contribute to TRS. One possibility is that, as patients spend longer in a psychotic state, the neural networks associated with psychosis are potentiated.

Our findings indicate that two distinct patterns of treatment resistance develop in patients, with the majority displaying treatment resistance from the onset and a smaller subset of patients developing treatment resistance after periods of relapse or with a later emergence of an intrinsic treatment resistance with a propensity for poorer outcomes and attenuated antipsychotic response over time.

Conclusions

TRS affects up to one-third of people with schizophrenia, with a population prevalence of 0.2%. TRS is associated with increased social and economic burden, and 80% of the total health and economic costs for schizophrenia are associated with TRS. TRS is associated with increased functional impairment compared to other refractory mental disorders, with high unemployment, lost productivity, high social impairment, and reduced quality of life. Several sociodemographic, clinical, and biological predictor variables have been assessed in relation to TRS, but there remains a lack of replicated findings to guide the prediction of TRS. However, emerging evidence indicates that early resistance to antipsychotics is a not uncommon phenomenon, with the majority of those with treatment resistance being resistant to non-clozapine antipsychotics from the time of illness onset. Earlier recognition and diagnosis of treatment resistance can lead to a more optimal use of clozapine with potential to improve clinical, functional, and social outcomes for people with TRS.

REFERENCES

Agid, O., Arenovich, T., Sajeev, G., et al. (2011). An algorithm-based approach to first-episode schizophrenia: response rates over 3 prospective antipsychotic trials with a retrospective data analysis. *Journal of Clinical Psychiatry*, 72, 1439–44.

Aitchison, K. J., Kerwin, R. W. (1997). Cost-effectiveness of clozapine. A UK clinic-based study. *Br J Psychiatry*, 171, 125–30.

Andrew A., Knapp, M., McCrone, P., Parsonage, M., Trachtenberg, M. (2012). *Effective Interventions in Schizophrenia: the economic case*. London: London School of Economics and Political Science.

Anttila, S., Illi, A., Kampman, O., Mattila, K. M., Lehtimaki, T., Leinonen, E. (2005). Lack of association between two polymorphisms of brain-derived neurotrophic factor and response to typical neuroleptics. *J Neural Transm (Vienna)*, 112, 885–90.

Anttila, S., Kampman, O., Illi, A., Rontu, R., Lehtimaki, T., Leinonen, E. (2007). Association between 5-HT2A, TPH1 and GNB3 genotypes and response to typical neuroleptics: a serotonergic approach. *BMC Psychiatry*, 7, 22.

Bachmann, C. J., Aagaard, L., Bernardo, M., et al. (2017). International trends in clozapine use: a study in 17 countries. *Acta Psychiatr Scand*, 136, 37–51.

Carbon, M., Correll, C. U. (2014). Clinical predictors of therapeutic response to antipsychotics in schizophrenia. *Dialogues in Clinical Neuroscience*, 16, 505–24.

Chouinard, G. (1991). Severe cases of neuroleptic-induced supersensitivity psychosis. Diagnostic criteria for the disorder and its treatment. *Schizophrenia Research*, 5, 21–33.

Chouinard, G., Chouinard, V. A. (2008). Atypical antipsychotics: CATIE study, drug-induced movement disorder and resulting iatrogenic psychiatric-like symptoms, supersensitivity rebound psychosis and withdrawal discontinuation syndromes. *Psychotherapy and Psychosomatics*, 77, 69–77.

Conley, R. R., Kelly, D. L. (2001). Management of treatment resistance in schizophrenia. *Biol Psychiatry*, 50, 898–911.

Davidson, M., Kapara, O., Goldberg, S., Yoffe, R., Noy, S., Weiser, M. (2016). A nation-wide study on the percentage of schizophrenia and bipolar disorder patients who earn minimum wage or above. *Schizophr Bull*, 42, 443–7.

Davies, L. M., Drummond, M. F. (1994). Economics and schizophrenia: the real cost. *Br J Psychiatry Suppl*, 25, 18–21.

Demjaha, A., Murray, R. M., Mcguire, P. K., Kapur, S., Howes, O. D. (2012). Dopamine synthesis capacity in patients with treatment-resistant schizophrenia. *Am J Psychiatry*, 169, 1203–10.

Demjaha, A., Egerton, A., Murray, R. M., et al. (2014). Antipsychotic treatment resistance in schizophrenia associated with elevated glutamate levels but normal dopamine function. *Biol Psychiatry*, 75, e11–e13.

Demjaha, A., Lappin, J. M., Stahl, D., et al. (2017). Antipsychotic treatment resistance in first-episode psychosis: prevalence, subtypes and predictors. *Psychol Med*, 47, 1981–9.

Egerton, A., Brugger, S., Raffin, M., et al. (2012). Anterior cingulate glutamate levels related to clinical status following treatment in first-episode schizophrenia. *Neuropsychopharmacology*, 37, 2515–21.

Emsley, R., Nuamah, I., Hough, D., Gopal, S. (2012). Treatment response after relapse in a placebo-controlled maintenance trial in schizophrenia. *Schizophrenia Research*, 138, 29–34.

Essock, S. M., Hargreaves, W. A., Covell, N. H., Goethe, J. (1996a). Clozapine's effectiveness for patients in state hospitals: results from a randomized trial. *Psychopharmacol Bull*, 32, 683–97.

Essock, S. M., Hargreaves, W. A., Dohm, F. A., Goethe, J., Carver, L., Hipshman, L. (1996b). Clozapine eligibility among state hospital patients. *Schizophr Bull,* 22, 15–25.

Frank, J., Lang, M., Witt, S. H. et al. (2015). Identification of increased genetic risk scores for schizophrenia in treatment-resistant patients. *Molecular Psychiatry,* 20, 150–1.

Gillespie, A. L., Samanaite, R., Mill, J., Egerton, A., Maccabe, J. H. (2017). Is treatment-resistant schizophrenia categorically distinct from treatment-responsive schizophrenia? A systematic review. *BMC Psychiatry,* 17, 12.

Goldberger, C., Gourion, D., Leroy, S., et al. (2005). Population-based and family-based association study of 5'UTR polymorphism of the reelin gene and schizophrenia. *Am J Med Genet B Neuropsychiatr Genet,* 137b, 51–5.

Goren, J. L., Rose, A. J., Smith, E. G., Ney, J. P. (2016). The business case for expanded clozapine utilization. *Psychiatr Serv,* 67, 1197–205.

Hayhurst, K. P., Brown, P., Lewis, S. W. (2002). The cost-effectiveness of clozapine: a controlled, population-based, mirror-image study. *J Psychopharmacol,* 16, 169–75.

Horsdal, H. T., Wimberley, T., Kohler-Forsberg, O., Baandrup, L., Gasse, C. (2017). Association between global functioning at first schizophrenia diagnosis and treatment resistance. *Early Interv Psychiatry,* doi: 10.1111/eip.12522. [Epub ahead of print].

Howes, O. D., Vergunst, F., Gee, S., Mcguire, P., Kapur, S., Taylor, D. (2012). Adherence to treatment guidelines in clinical practice: study of antipsychotic treatment prior to clozapine initiation. *Br J Psychiatry,* 201, 481–5.

Howes, O. D., Mccutcheon, R., Agid, O., et al. (2017). Treatment-resistant schizophrenia: Treatment Response and Resistance in Psychosis (TRRIP) Working Group Consensus Guidelines on Diagnosis and Terminology. *Am J Psychiatry,* 174, 216–29.

Iasevoli, F., Giordano, S., Balletta, R., et al. (2016). Treatment resistant schizophrenia is associated with the worst community functioning among severely-ill highly-disabling psychiatric conditions and is the most relevant predictor of poorer achievements in functional milestones. *Prog Neuropsychopharmacol Biol Psychiatry,* 65, 34–48.

Inada, T., Nakamura, A., Iijima, Y. (2003). Relationship between catechol-O-methyltransferase polymorphism and treatment-resistant schizophrenia. *Am J Med Genet B Neuropsychiatr Genet,* 120b, 35–9.

Iyo, M., Tadokoro, S., Kanahara, N., et al. (2013). Optimal extent of dopamine D2 receptor occupancy by antipsychotics for treatment of dopamine supersensitivity psychosis and late-onset psychosis. *J Clin Psychopharmacol,* 33, 398–404.

Jaaskelainen, E., Juola, P., Hirvonen, N., et al. (2013). A systematic review and meta-analysis of recovery in schizophrenia. *Schizophr Bull,* 39, 1296–306.

Ji, X., Takahashi, N., Saito, S., et al. (2008). Relationship between three serotonin receptor subtypes (HTR3A, HTR2A and HTR4) and treatment-resistant schizophrenia in the Japanese population. *Neurosci Lett,* 435, 95–8.

Joober, R., Benkelfat, C., Brisebois, K., et al. (1999). T102C polymorphism in the *5HT2A* gene and schizophrenia: relation to phenotype and drug response variability. *J Psychiatry Neurosci,* 24, 141–6.

Juarez-Reyes, M. G., Shumway, M., Battle, C., Bacchetti, P., Hansen, M. S., Hargreaves, W. A. (1995). Effects of stringent criteria on eligibility for clozapine among public mental health clients. *Psychiatr Serv,* 46, 801–6.

Kane, J., Honigfeld, G., Singer, J., Meltzer, H. (1988). Clozapine for the treatment-resistant schizophrenic. A double-blind comparison with chlorpromazine. Arch Gen Psychiatry, 45, 789–96.

Kennedy, J. L., Altar, C. A., Taylor, D. L., Degtiar, I., Hornberger, J. C. (2014). The social and economic burden of treatment-resistant schizophrenia: a systematic literature review. Int Clin Psychopharmacol, 29, 63–76.

Kirov, G., Pocklington, A. J., Holmans, P., et al. (2012). De novo CNV analysis implicates specific abnormalities of postsynaptic signalling complexes in the pathogenesis of schizophrenia. Mol Psychiatry, 17, 142–53.

Kirwan, P., O'Connor, L., Sharma, K., McDonald, C. (2017). The impact of switching to clozapine on psychiatric hospital admissions: a mirror-image study. Irish Journal of Psychological Medicine, doi.org/10.1017/ipm.2017.28.

Knapp, M., Mangalore, R. & Simon, J. (2004). The global costs of schizophrenia. Schizophr Bull, 30, 279–93.

Kolakowska, T., Williams, A. O., Ardern, M., et al. (1985). Schizophrenia with good and poor outcome. I: Early clinical features, response to neuroleptics and signs of organic dysfunction. Br J Psychiatry, 146, 229–39.

Krebs, M. O., Guillin, O., Bourdell, M. C., et al. (2000). Brain derived neurotrophic factor (BDNF) gene variants association with age at onset and therapeutic response in schizophrenia. Mol Psychiatry, 5, 558–62.

Krebs, M. O., Sautel, F., Bourdel, M. C., et al. (1998). Dopamine D3 receptor gene variants and substance abuse in schizophrenia. Mol Psychiatry, 3, 337–41.

Lahdelma, L., Ahokas, A., Andersson, L. C., et al. (1998). Association between HLA-A1 allele and schizophrenia gene(s) in patients refractory to conventional neuroleptics but responsive to clozapine medication. Tissue Antigens, 51, 200–3.

Lally, J., Maccabe, J. H. (2015). Antipsychotic medication in schizophrenia: a review. Br Med Bull, 114, 169–79.

Lally, J., Ajnakina, O., Di Forti, M., et al. (2016a). Two distinct patterns of treatment resistance: clinical predictors of treatment resistance in first-episode schizophrenia spectrum psychoses. Psychol Med, 46, 3231–40.

Lally, J., Gaughran, F., Timms, P., Curran, S. R. (2016b). Treatment-resistant schizophrenia: current insights on the pharmacogenomics of antipsychotics. Pharmgenomics Pers Med, 9, 117–29.

Lally, J., Ajnakina, O., Stubbs, B., et al. (2017). Remission and recovery from first-episode psychosis in adults: systematic review and meta-analysis of long-term outcome studies. Br J Psychiatry, 211, 350–8.

Land, R., Siskind, D., McCardle, P., Kisely, S., Winckel, K., Hollingworth, S. A. (2017). The impact of clozapine on hospital use: a systematic review and meta-analysis. Acta Psychiatr Scand, 135, 296–309.

Lewis, S. W., Barnes, T. R., Davies, L., et al. (2006). Randomized controlled trial of effect of prescription of clozapine versus other second-generation antipsychotic drugs in resistant schizophrenia. Schizophr Bull, 32, 715–23.

Lin, C. C., Wang, Y. C., Chen, J. Y., et al. (2008). Artificial neural network prediction of clozapine response with combined pharmacogenetic and clinical data. Comput Methods Programs Biomed, 91, 91–9.

Mangalore, R., Knapp, M. (2007). Cost of schizophrenia in England. *J Ment Health Policy Econ*, 10, 23–41.

Martin, A. K., Mowry, B. (2016). Increased rare duplication burden genomewide in patients with treatment-resistant schizophrenia. *Psychological Medicine*, 46, 469–76.

Marwaha, S., Johnson, S., Bebbington, P., et al. (2007). Rates and correlates of employment in people with schizophrenia in the UK, France and Germany. *Br J Psychiatry*, 191, 30–7.

McCutcheon, R., Beck, K., D'Ambrosio, E., et al. (2018). Antipsychotic plasma levels in the assessment of poor treatment response in schizophrenia. *Acta Psychiatr Scand*, 137, 39–46.

McGrath, J., Saha, S., Chant, D., Welham, J. (2008). Schizophrenia: a concise overview of incidence, prevalence, and mortality. *Epidemiol Rev*, 30, 67–76.

Meged, S., Stein, D., Sitrota, P., et al. (1999). Human leukocyte antigen typing, response to neuroleptics, and clozapine-induced agranulocytosis in jewish Israeli schizophrenic patients. *Int Clin Psychopharmacol*, 14, 305–12.

Meltzer, H. Y. (1997). Treatment-resistant schizophrenia—the role of clozapine. *Curr Med Res Opin*, 14, 1–20.

Meltzer, H. Y., Rabinowitz, J., Lee, M. A., et al. (1997). Age at onset and gender of schizophrenic patients in relation to neuroleptic resistance. *Am J Psychiatry*, 154, 475–82.

Menezes, N. M., Arenovich, T., Zipursky, R. B. (2006). A systematic review of longitudinal outcome studies of first-episode psychosis. *Psychol Med*, 36, 1349–62.

Miller, B. J., Buckley, P., Seabolt, W., Mellor, A., Kirkpatrick, B. (2011). Meta-analysis of cytokine alterations in schizophrenia: clinical status and antipsychotic effects. *Biol Psychiatry*, 70, 663–71.

Mortimer, A. M., Singh, P., Shepherd, C. J., Puthiryackal, J. (2010). Clozapine for treatment-resistant schizophrenia: National Institute of Clinical Excellence (NICE) guidance in the real world. *Clin Schizophr Relat Psychoses*, 4, 49–55.

NICE. (2014). *Psychosis and Schizophrenia in Adults: treatment and management (Clinical guideline 178)*. London: Royal College of Psychiatrists.

Ortiz, B. B., Araujo Filho, G. M., Araripe Neto, A. G., Medeiros, D., Bressan, R. A. (2013). Is disorganized schizophrenia a predictor of treatment resistance? Evidence from an observational study. *Revista Brasileira de Psiquiatria*, 35, 432–4.

Palmer, B. A., Pankratz, V. S., Bostwick, J. M. (2005). The lifetime risk of suicide in schizophrenia: a reexamination. *Arch Gen Psychiatry*, 62, 247–53.

Robinson, D. G., Woerner, M. G., Alvir, J. M., et al. (1999). Predictors of treatment response from a first episode of schizophrenia or schizoaffective disorder. *Am J Psychiatry*, 156, 544–9.

Schennach, R., Riedel, M., Musil, R., Moller, H. J. (2012). Treatment response in first-episode schizophrenia. *Clin Psychopharmacol Neurosci*, 10, 78–87.

Schizophrenia Working Group of the Psychiatric Genomics Consortium. (2014). Biological insights from 108 schizophrenia-associated genetic loci. *Nature*, 511, 421–7.

Simeone, J. C., Ward, A. J., Rotella, P., Collins, J., Windisch, R. (2015). An evaluation of variation in published estimates of schizophrenia prevalence from 1990 horizontal line 2013: a systematic literature review. *BMC Psychiatry*, 15, 193.

CHAPTER 4

Stroup, T. S., Gerhard, T., Crystal, S., Huang, C., Olfson, M. (2016). Comparative effectiveness of clozapine and standard antipsychotic treatment in adults with schizophrenia. *Am J Psychiatry*, 173, 166–73.

Taipale, H., Mehtala, J., Tanskanen, A., Tiihonen, J. (2017). Comparative effectiveness of antipsychotic drugs for rehospitalization in schizophrenia—a nationwide study with 20-year follow-up. *Schizophr Bull*, doi: 10.1093/schbul/sbx176. [Epub ahead of print].

Taylor, D. L., Tiwari, A. K., Lieberman, J. A., et al. (2016). Genetic association analysis of N-methyl-d-aspartate receptor subunit gene *GRIN2B* and clinical response to clozapine. *Human Psychopharmacology: Clinical and Experimental*, 31, 121–34.

Terkelsen, K. G., Grosser, R. C. (1990). Estimating clozapine's cost to the nation. *Hosp Community Psychiatry*, 41, 863–9.

Vanelle, J. M. (1995). [Treatment refractory schizophrenia]. *L'Encephale*, 21 Spec No 3, 13–21.

Vanelle, J. M., Olie, J. P., Levy-Soussan, P. (1994). New antipsychotics in schizophrenia: the French experience. *Acta Psychiatrica Scandinavica Suppl*, 380, 59–63.

Wheeler, A., Humberstone, V., Robinson, G. (2009). Outcomes for schizophrenia patients with clozapine treatment: how good does it get? *J Psychopharmacol*, 23, 957–65.

WHO. (2001). *The World Health Report 2001: Mental Health: New Understanding, New Hope*. Geneva: World Health Organization.

Wiersma, D., Nienhuis, F. J., Slooff, C. J., Giel, R. (1998). Natural course of schizophrenic disorders: a 15-year followup of a Dutch incidence cohort. *Schizophr Bull*, 24, 75–85.

Wimberley, T., Pedersen, C. B., Maccabe, J. H., et al. (2016a). Inverse association between urbanicity and treatment resistance in schizophrenia. *Schizophr Res*, 174, 150–5.

Wimberley, T., Støvring, H., Sørensen, H. J., Horsdal, H. T., Maccabe, J. H., Gasse, C. (2016b). Predictors of treatment resistance in patients with schizophrenia: a population-based cohort study. *The Lancet Psychiatry*, 3, 358–66.

Zhang, J. P., Lencz, T., Geisler, S., Derosse, P., Bromet, E. J., Malhotra, A. K. (2013). Genetic variation in BDNF is associated with antipsychotic treatment resistance in patients with schizophrenia. *Schizophr Res*, 146, 285–8.

CHAPTER 5

The neurobiology of antipsychotic treatment response and resistance

Stephen J. Kaar, Steven Potkin, and Oliver Howes

KEY POINTS

- The first antipsychotic drugs were discovered as a result of serendipity and careful clinical observation, long before dopamine was established as a neurotransmitter.

- All currently licensed antipsychotic drugs block a substantial proportion of dopamine D2/3 receptors at clinically effective doses.

- Imaging studies in patients have shown that there is a therapeutic window for dopamine D2/3 receptor blockade by antipsychotic drugs that balances efficacy with risk of side effects.

- Several lines of evidence indicate that the neurobiology of treatment resistance does not involve the same alterations in dopamine function seen in the majority of patients.

- Clozapine's preferential action at D1 and serotonin 2A receptors has focused attention on targeting these receptors as therapeutic strategies for treatment resistance.

The determinants of treatment response

A number of antipsychotics still in common use today, such as chlorpromazine, clozapine, and haloperidol, were discovered before dopamine was recognized as a neurotransmitter in its own right, and before the discovery of dopamine receptors. Rodent studies in the 1960s showed that antipsychotics altered levels of dopamine and its metabolites, indicating that they affected the dopamine system (Carlsson and Lindqvist, 1963; Ross and Renyi, 1967; Glowinski and Iversen, 1966). These were followed by in-vitro binding studies in the 1970s, which demonstrated that the clinical potency of antipsychotic drugs correlated with their affinity for dopamine receptors (Creese et al., 1976; Seeman and Lee, 1975; Seeman et al., 1975; 1976).

Molecular cloning studies subsequently showed that there are five dopamine receptors in humans (Seeman, 2001). These are expressed as two main subtypes: the D2-like family, comprising D2, D3, and D4 receptors, and the D1-like family, comprising D1 and D5 receptors (Spano et al., 1978; Kebabian and Calne, 1979). In the

1980s molecular neuroimaging techniques, such as single photon emission computed tomography (SPECT) and positron emission tomography (PET), started to be applied to investigate dopamine receptor occupancy by antipsychotic drugs in vivo in patients. These techniques showed that antipsychotic drugs block striatal dopamine D2/3 receptors in vivo, and indicate that substantial blockade, generally greater than 50% of D2/3 receptors, is required for a high likelihood of a clinically significant response (Kapur et al., 1997; 1999; 2000; Richtand et al., 2007; Brucke et al., 1992; Pilowsky et al., 1993; Nyberg et al., 1995). However, these studies also showed that D2/3 receptor occupancy greater than about 80% was generally associated with little additional clinical benefit but with an increased risk of extrapyramidal side effects and hyperprolactinaemia (Kapur et al., 2000), indicating that there is a therapeutic window for dopamine D2/3 receptor blockade by antipsychotic drugs, with receptor occupancy of between roughly 60% and 80% optimizing the chance of response whilst minimizing the risk of D2/3 receptor mediated side effects. Lurasidone is a second-generation antipsychotic medication approved for the treatment of schizophrenia over a dose range of 40–160 mg/day. The relationship between lurasidone dose, dopamine D2 receptor (D2R) occupancy, and clinical efficacy provides an example of these principles. Blood lurasidone concentration, but not dose, is significantly correlated with D2/3R occupancy, and D2/3R occupancy is associated with positive but not negative symptom improvement or the presence of movement symptoms. Greater than 65% D2/3R occupancy is generally achieved across the clinical dose range of 80–160 mg/day, but some patients require higher doses to achieve sufficient D2/3R occupancy to obtain adequate clinical response: non-responders to 80 mg/day randomized to 160 mg/day showed greater improvement than those randomized to remain on 80 mg/day (Potkin et al., 2014; Loebel et al., 2013; 2016).

However, whilst such studies indicate how antipsychotic drugs work, they do not explain why they work. Molecular imaging studies in antipsychotic-naïve patients show that D2/3 receptor availability is unaltered at the onset of psychosis (Howes et al., 2012), which suggests that dopamine receptor alterations do not explain the disorder or why antipsychotics work, at least in the initial stages of the disease. However, alterations in aspects of presynaptic dopaminergic activity are present at illness onset. Specifically, increased dopamine synthesis capacity is seen in people with prodromal signs of psychosis, and is linked to the subclinical psychotic symptoms (Howes et al., 2009; 2011). Moreover, in patients with established schizophrenia, PET and SPECT studies have found greater striatal dopamine synthesis and release capacity relative to matched controls, with a large effect size of about 0.8 (Howes et al., 2012), and greater dopamine release capacity has been associated with a greater induction of psychotic symptoms. Thus, in schizophrenia the major disturbance in the dopamine system appears to be presynaptic, with excess dopamine synthesis and release capacity underlying the development of psychosis. This explains why antipsychotic drugs are effective because they dampen the consequences of dysregulated dopamine synthesis and release by blocking the D2/3 receptors.

The biology of pseudo-treatment resistance

Pseudo-treatment resistance describes circumstances where a patient's condition appears to be resistant to treatment but, in fact, there is insufficient drug at the target site for a response e.g. lurasidone example above. To reach its target, D2/3 receptors in the brain, an orally administered antipsychotic drug has to undergo a number of processes: ingestion and absorption from the gut, first and second pass metabolism, transit across the blood–brain barrier, biodistribution throughout the brain without being excluded by the P-glycoprotein transporter (P-gp) as is the case with risperidone, and, finally, binding to dopamine receptors. A disturbance in any one of these processes may affect the final degree of dopamine receptor blockade achieved.

Clearly, oral drugs that are not ingested are unable to act. Non-concordance with prescribed medication is a huge problem across clinical medicine, and this is also true in the treatment of schizophrenia, where reduced insight, cognitive impairments, and stigma affect adherence (Chakrabarti, 2014; Haddad et al., 2014). Careful clinical assessment that encourages patient engagement with treatment, the use of other sources of information (medical notes, opinions of carers and relatives), and, if available, drug plasma level testing can be helpful in assessing adherence (Horvitz-Lennon et al., 2017). If a patient struggles to remember to take medication then memory aids such as electronic reminders, medication boxes, and establishing a regular routine can be helpful (Cramer and Rosenheck, 1999). If these are ineffective, then long-acting injectable preparations are recommended.

However, it is important to recognize that a proportion of patients show rapid metabolism of antipsychotic drugs such that, even with good concordance, inadequate levels of drug reach the target site (Horvitz-Lennon et al., 2017). Rapid metabolism can be due to patients carrying genetic variants affecting liver enzymes that metabolize antipsychotics. These are surprisingly common, being present in about 5–10% of the population, depending on the variant (Dahl, 2002). Genetic tests to identify variants affecting metabolism have been developed, although they are not yet widely available in clinical practice. In addition to genetic variants affecting metabolism of antipsychotic drugs, cytochrome P450 enzyme inducers such as tobacco and other medications (e.g. carbamazepine) can significantly increase metabolism of drugs and thereby reduce plasma antipsychotic levels and lead to poor treatment response (De Leon, 2004; Kennedy et al., 2013).

Patients in these categories may thus require higher doses of antipsychotic to reach adequate D2 occupancy levels (see the discussion of lurasidone in the section on 'Determinants of treatment response'). In routine clinical practice, where molecular imaging and detailed pharmacokinetic analysis are not available, this may justify an empirical trial of an antipsychotic at a high dose, although this should be carefully evaluated and form the exception rather than the rule (see Chapter 9).

The biology of primary treatment resistance

Molecular imaging studies show that some patients fail to respond to antipsychotic drug treatment despite the drug blocking a substantial proportion of striatal D2/3 receptors (Wolkin et al., 1989; Pilowsky et al., 1993). These findings indicate that, whilst D2/3 receptor occupancy is necessary for antipsychotic drug action, it is not sufficient in all patients.

What, then, underlies psychosis in these patients? One possibility is that, in such cases, psychosis is not due to dopaminergic dysfunction at all. In line with this, it has been hypothesized that schizophrenia has at least two neuro-chemical subtypes: a type A subtype characterized by hyperdopaminergia and good response to antipsychotics, and a type B subtype characterized by normal dopamine function that shows little response to dopamine receptor blockade because the psychosis is due to abnormalities in other systems (Howes and Kapur, 2014).

Experiments measuring dopamine metabolite levels in patients with schizo-phrenia tend to show a bimodal distribution; one group has elevated levels, the other relatively normal levels (Ottong and Garver, 1997; Yoshimura et al., 2003). Interestingly, those patients who show higher baseline plasma homovanillic acid (pHVA) levels, the major metabolite of dopamine, are more likely to respond to antipsychotic treatment (Chang et al., 1990; 1993; Yoshimura et al., 2003). Moreover, a greater reduction in pHVA levels has been associated with greater response to antipsychotic treatment (Baeza et al., 2009). It appears, therefore, that patients who show the greatest reduction in pHVA levels tend to be the ones who respond to treatment (Davidson et al., 1991). Conversely, non-responders tend to be the patients who show normal or reduced levels of dopamine metab-olites at baseline, and less change with antipsychotic treatment (Heritch, 1990; Karoum et al., 1987). When variability in pHVA concentrations is measured, greater variability is associated with positive symptoms and a greater decrease in symptoms following antipsychotic treatment (Zumárraga et al., 2011).

Post-mortem findings in patients with schizophrenia are not clear-cut, po-tentially because the effect of lifetime antipsychotic medication on D2Rs cre-ates a significant confounding effect (Seeman et al., 1987; Davis et al., 1991). Notwithstanding this, patients who responded to antipsychotic treatment tended to have a higher density of dopamine synapses than non-responders in one post-mortem series (Roberts et al., 2009).

PET studies have provided molecular imaging evidence to support the idea of a differing brain dopamine pathophysiology in treatment-resistant schizophrenia. Again, presynaptic dopamine dysfunction appears to be key as PET studies that measure dopamine synthesis capacity suggest that patients who fail to respond to antipsychotic treatment lack the elevated dopamine synthesis capacity that is seen in patients who respond to antipsychotic treatment (Demjaha et al., 2012; Jauhar et al., 2018). Such findings support the hypothesis that hyperdopaminergia is associated with the positive symptoms of schizophrenia and treatment response, whereas non-response is associated with an absence of hyperdopaminergia.

So, if not dopamine, which other neurotransmitters may contribute to psychosis in these patients? One leading candidate is glutamatergic dysregulation. Glutamate is the major excitatory neurotransmitter in the brain (Rothman et al., 2003), and abnormal glutamatergic neurotransmission has been considered as a potential neurobiological mechanism underlying schizophrenia pathogenesis for decades (Howes et al., 2015; Kim et al., 1980, Krystal et al., 1994; Stone et al., 2007). The psychotomimetic effects of non-competitive glutamate receptor antagonists such as phencyclidine (PCP) and ketamine adds further weight to the evidence for glutamatergic abnormalities having a role in psychosis, in particular because such drugs induce psychotic symptoms that appear to closely mimic those seen in schizophrenia in healthy controls (Krystal et al., 1994) and induce positive symptoms of schizophrenia in patients (Lahti et al., 1995). Ketamine also increases amphetamine-induced dopamine release in healthy controls, which adds weight to the hypothesis that impaired glutamatergic regulation of dopamine may explain the increases in amphetamine-induced dopamine release in schizophrenia (Kegeles et al., 2000).

Magnetic resonance spectroscopy (MRS) allows the concentration of neurochemicals to be indexed in vivo within the brain, and a large recent meta-analysis of MRS studies showed elevation of glutamatergic metabolites across several brain regions in schizophrenia (Merritt et al., 2016). Studies using this technique conducted in patients whose illness has shown a poor response to antipsychotics, including patients meeting fairly rigorous criteria for treatment resistance, have shown that levels of glutamate and its metabolite glutamine are elevated in at least some brain regions when compared with levels in patients whose illness has shown a good response to antipsychotic treatment (Egerton et al., 2012; Demjaha et al., 2014; Mouchlianitis et al., 2016). However, other findings indicate that levels of glutamate may be reduced in patients who show a response to antipsychotic treatment, but not markedly change in patients who do not respond (De La Fuente-Sandoval et al., 2013). Thus, the picture could be more complicated than a categorical distinction between illness subtypes, and it remains possible that glutamatergic differences are secondary to other neurobiological alterations rather than the primary pathophysiology underlying treatment-resistant psychosis.

The indolamines, such as lysergic acid diethylamide (LSD), can induce psychotic symptoms, such as hallucinations, similar to those seen in schizophrenia. They are partial agonists at the 5-HT2a receptor. Partly as a consequence, 5-HT2a receptor antagonists such as ritanserin have been evaluated as treatments for schizophrenia. Adjunctive ritanserin improved symptoms in schizophrenia patients treated with haloperidol, improving both positive and negative symptoms while decreasing motor side effects (Duinkerke et al., 1993). The results seen with adjunctive ritanserin provided the foundation for the development of the antipsychotic risperidone, a potent antagonist of D2 and 5-HT2a receptors.

Patients with schizophrenia who received monotherapy with M100907, a selective 5-HT2a antagonist devoid of dopaminergic activity, showed a statistically significant improvement relative to placebo on the Positive And Negative Syndrome Scale (PANSS) and Clinical Global Impression (CGI) scale in a large randomized clinical trial (personal communication, S. G. Potkin). In a recent study in patients with an acute exacerbation of schizophrenia (Meltzer et al., 2012), adjunctive pimavanserin, a selective 5-HT2a antagonist, enhanced the efficacy of low-dose (2 mg daily) risperidone, achieving comparable efficacy to 6 mg/day risperidone with fewer side effects. Post-mortem studies provide additional evidence for 5-HT2a alterations in schizophrenia, showing reductions with a large effect size (Selvaraj et al., 2014). These lines of evidence suggest that 5-HT2a alterations may contribute to the pathophysiology of treatment resistance. The potential role of adjunctive pimavanserin for augmenting dopamine D2/3 blockers to treat schizophrenia is now being evaluated in ongoing phase 3 trials.

The pharmacology of clozapine may also provide clues to the biology of treatment resistance. It has a relatively low affinity for dopamine D2/3 receptors compared to most other antipsychotic drugs. Whilst it does block an appreciable proportion in vivo at clinically effective doses, its D2/3 occupancy is also lower than most other antipsychotics, probably partly reflecting its fast kinetics as well as its relatively low D2/3R affinity (Kessler et al., 2006; Kapur and Seeman, 2001). Clozapine has a relatively high affinity for serotonin 2a receptors. At one time this was thought to contribute to its superior efficacy (Meltzer, 1989), although subsequent in-vivo imaging studies have suggested that serotonin 2a receptor occupancy is unlikely to account for the therapeutic efficacy of current antipsychotic drugs (Kapur et al., 1998; Kapur and Seeman, 2001). Clozapine also has a relatively high affinity for dopamine D1 receptors, and shows higher D1 occupancy than most other antipsychotics at therapeutic doses (Nordstrom et al., 1995). Moreover, D1 receptor polymorphisms have been found to predict clinical response to clozapine (Potkin et al., 2003). This suggests that, whilst it is not clear if D1 receptors are altered specifically in patients with treatment-resistant schizophrenia, D1 antagonism may be a potential mechanism to treat resistant symptoms. This is now being evaluated in phase 3 clinical trials of a novel drug, Lu AF35700, that has higher affinity for D1 receptors over D2 receptors (see Chapter 14).

The biology of secondary treatment resistance

A proportion of patients show a good initial response to antipsychotic treatment but over time response becomes inadequate; this is manifested as breakthrough symptoms or poor response to re-starting antipsychotic treatment after a relapse, for example (see Chapter 4 for further discussion). The clinical picture suggests that psychosis in these individuals is related to dopamine dysfunction (fitting into subtype A in the nomenclature), but that adaptive changes occur in response to prolonged antipsychotic treatment, or, given that patients often stop and re-start treatment, with intermittent treatment. What are these changes that could account for the development of treatment resistance?

One possibility is the development of dopamine supersensitivity (Seeman, 2013) secondary to long-term treatment with D2 antagonists. Long-term treatment with antipsychotic medication is associated with higher D2/3 receptor availability, at least in some patients (Silvestri et al., 2000). Thus, upregulation in D2/3 receptor levels with treatment could mean that a given antipsychotic dose is no longer sufficient to block dopaminergic neurotransmission adequately, leading to breakthrough symptoms (Chouinard and Chouinard, 2008). A related possibility is that there is an increase in the proportion of dopamine D2 receptors with a high affinity for dopamine (Samaha et al., 2007), potentially making the dopaminergic system become supersensitive to dopamine release.

Another, related, possibility is that it is not the antipsychotic treatment but other factors that lead to dopaminergic supersensitivity. This is suggested by evidence that patients with schizophrenia who are dependent on substances show blunted dopamine release relative to controls but, nevertheless, dopamine release is associated with the induction of psychotic symptoms in these individuals, suggesting that they show heightened sensitivity to dopamine release (Thompson et al., 2013).

These possibilities are not mutually exclusive, of course, and could explain the clinical observation that patients who have been on long-term treatment sometimes require higher doses of antipsychotic treatment than first-episode patients (Remington and Kapur, 2010). Longitudinal studies are required to test these theories out and to determine why this might occur in some but not all patients.

Conclusions

The dopamine system is central both to the neurobiology of psychosis in the majority of patients with schizophrenia and to the therapeutic action of antipsychotic drugs, with the potential exception of clozapine. Recent findings have refined our understanding of the nature of the dopaminergic alterations in the disorder by identifying elevated dopamine synthesis and release capacity as the major locus underlying psychosis in most patients. However, whilst dopamine D2/3 receptor blockade is critical for therapeutic response with antipsychotics, a significant number of patients do not respond despite adequate dopamine D2/3 receptor blockade. Such patients do not seem to show the same dopaminergic changes as seen in the majority of patients with schizophrenia. Their illness may, instead, be linked to more marked glutamatergic alterations, which may explain why dopamine receptor blockade is ineffective. In other patients, the secondary effects of long-term treatment, such as dopamine D2/3 receptor upregulation, may lead to the development of treatment resistance.

CHAPTER 5

REFERENCES

Baeza, I., Castro-Fornieles, J., Deulofeu, R., et al. (2009). Plasma homovanillic acid differences in clinical subgroups of first episode schizophrenic patients. Psychiatry Res, 168, 110–18.

Brucke, T., Roth, J., Podreka, I., Strobl, R., Wenger, S., Asenbaum, S. (1992). Striatal dopamine D2-receptor blockade by typical and atypical neuroleptics. Lancet, 339, 497.

Carlsson, A., Lindqvist, M. (1963). Effect of chlorpromazine or haloperidol on formation of 3-methoxytyramine and normetanephrine in mouse brain. Acta Pharmacologica Toxicologica, 20, 140–4.

Chakrabarti, S. (2014). What's in a name? Compliance, adherence and concordance in chronic psychiatric disorders. World J Psychiatry, 4, 30–6.

Chang, W. H., Chen, T. Y., Lin, S. K., et al. (1990). Plasma catecholamine metabolites in schizophrenics: evidence for the two-subtype concept. Biol Psychiatry, 27, 510–18.

Chang, W. H., Hwu, H. G., Chen, T. Y., et al. (1993). Plasma homovanillic acid and treatment response in a large group of schizophrenic patients. Schizophr Res, 10, 259–65.

Chouinard, G., Chouinard, V. A. (2008). Atypical antipsychotics: CATIE study, drug-induced movement disorder and resulting iatrogenic psychiatric-like symptoms, supersensitivity rebound psychosis and withdrawal discontinuation syndromes. Psychother Psychosom, 77, 69–77.

Cramer, J. A., Rosenheck, R. (1999). Enhancing medication compliance for people with serious mental illness. J Nerv Ment Dis, 187, 53–5.

Creese, I., Burt, D. R., Snyder, S. H. (1976). Dopamine receptor binding predicts clinical and pharmacological potencies of antischizophrenic drugs. Science, 192, 481–3.

Dahl, M. L. (2002). Cytochrome p450 phenotyping/genotyping in patients receiving antipsychotics: useful aid to prescribing? Clin Pharmacokinet, 41, 453–70.

Davidson, M., Kahn, R. S., Knott, P., et al. (1991). Effects of neuroleptic treatment on symptoms of schizophrenia and plasma homovanillic acid concentrations. Arch Gen Psychiatry, 48, 910–13.

Davis, K. L., Kahn, R. S., Ko, G., Davidson, M. (1991). Dopamine in schizophrenia: a review and reconceptualization. Am J Psychiatry, 148, 1474–86.

De La Fuente-Sandoval, C., León-Ortiz, P., Azcárraga, M., et al. (2013). Glutamate levels in the associative striatum before and after 4 weeks of antipsychotic treatment in first-episode psychosis: a longitudinal proton magnetic resonance spectroscopy study. JAMA Psychiatry, 70, 1057–66.

De Leon, J. (2004). Atypical antipsychotic dosing: the effect of smoking and caffeine. Psychiatr Serv, 55, 491–3.

Demjaha, A., Murray, R. M., McGuire, P. K., Kapur, S., Howes, O. D. (2012). Dopamine synthesis capacity in patients with treatment-resistant schizophrenia. Am J Psychiatry, 169, 1203–10.

Demjaha, A., Egerton, A., Murray, R. M., et al. (2014). Antipsychotic treatment resistance in schizophrenia associated with elevated glutamate levels but normal dopamine function. Biol Psychiatry, 75, e11–e13.

Duinkerke, S. J., Botter, P. A., Jansen, A. A., et al. (1993). Ritanserin, a selective 5-HT2/1C antagonist, and negative symptoms in schizophrenia. A placebo-controlled double-blind trial. Br J Psychiatry, 163, 451–5.

Egerton, A., Brugger, S., Raffin, M., et al. (2012). Anterior cingulate glutamate levels related to clinical status following treatment in first-episode schizophrenia. *Neuropsychopharmacology*, 37, 2515–21.

Glowinski, J., Iversen, L. L. (1966). Regional studies of catecholamines in the rat brain-I: the disposition of [3h]norepinephrine, [3h]dopamine and [3h]dopa in various regions of the brain. *J Neurochem*, 13, 655–69.

Haddad, P. M., Brain, C., Scott, J. (2014). Nonadherence with antipsychotic medication in schizophrenia: challenges and management strategies. *Patient Relat Outcome Meas*, 5, 43–62.

Heritch, A. J. (1990). Evidence for reduced and dysregulated turnover of dopamine in schizophrenia. *Schizophr Bull*, 16, 605–15.

Horvitz-Lennon, M., Mattke, S., Predmore, Z., Howes, O. D. (2017). The role of antipsychotic plasma levels in the treatment of schizophrenia. *Am J Psychiatry*, 174, 421–6.

Howes, O. D., Kapur, S. (2014). A neurobiological hypothesis for the classification of schizophrenia: type a (hyperdopaminergic) and type b (normodopaminergic). *Br J Psychiatry*, 205, 1–3.

Howes, O. D., Montgomery, A. J., Asselin, M. C., et al. (2009). Elevated striatal dopamine function linked to prodromal signs of schizophrenia. *Arch Gen Psychiatry*, 66, 13–20.

Howes, O. D., Bose, S. K., Turkheimer, F., et al. (2011). Dopamine synthesis capacity before onset of psychosis: a prospective [18F]-DOPA PET imaging study. *Am J Psychiatry*, 168, 1311–17.

Howes, O. D., Kambeitz, J., Kim, E., et al. (2012). The nature of dopamine dysfunction in schizophrenia and what this means for treatment. *Arch Gen Psychiatry*, 69, 776–86.

Howes, O., McCutcheon, R., Stone, J. (2015). Glutamate and dopamine in schizophrenia: an update for the 21st century. *J Psychopharmacol*, 29, 97–115.

Jauhar, S., Veronese, M., Nour, M. M., et al. (2018). Determinants of treatment response in first-episode psychosis: an 18F-DOPA PET study. *Mol Psychiatry*. doi: 10.1038/s-41380-018-0042-4. [Epub ahead of print]

Kapur, S., Seeman, P. (2001). Does fast dissociation from the dopamine D2 receptor explain the action of atypical antipsychotics?: a new hypothesis. *Am J Psychiatry*, 158, 360–9.

Kapur, S., Zipursky, R., Roy, P., et al. (1997). The relationship between D2 receptor occupancy and plasma levels on low dose oral haloperidol: a PET study. *Psychopharmacology (Berl)*, 131, 148–52.

Kapur, S., Zipursky, R. B., Remington, G., et al. (1998). 5-HT2 and D2 Receptor occupancy of olanzapine in schizophrenia: a PET investigation. *Am J Psychiatry*, 155, 921–8.

Kapur, S., Zipursky, R. B., Remington, G. (1999). Clinical and theoretical implications of 5-HT2 and D2 receptor occupancy of clozapine, risperidone, and olanzapine in schizophrenia. *Am J Psychiatry*, 156, 286–93.

Kapur, S., Zipursky, R., Jones, C., Remington, G., Houle, S. (2000). Relationship between dopamine D2 occupancy, clinical response, and side effects: a double-blind PET study of first-episode schizophrenia. *Am J Psychiatry*, 157, 514–20.

CHAPTER 5

Karoum, F., Karson, C. N., Bigelow, L. B., Lawson, W. B., Wyatt, R. (1987). Preliminary evidence of reduced combined output of dopamine and its metabolites in chronic schizophrenia. *Arch Gen Psychiatry*, 44, 604–7.

Kebabian, J. W., Calne, D. B. (1979). Multiple receptors for dopamine. *Nature*, 277, 93–6.

Kegeles, L. S., Abi-Dargham, A., Zea-Ponce, Y., et al. (2000). Modulation of amphetamine-induced striatal dopamine release by ketamine in humans: implications for schizophrenia. *Biol Psychiatry*, 48, 627–40.

Kennedy, W. K., Jann, M. W., Kutscher, E. C. (2013). Clinically significant drug interactions with atypical antipsychotics. *CNS Drugs*, 27, 1021–48.

Kessler, R. M., Ansari, M. S., Riccardi, P., et al. (2006). Occupancy of striatal and extrastriatal dopamine D2 receptors by clozapine and quetiapine. *Neuropsychopharmacology*, 31, 1991.

Kim, J. S., Kornhuber, H. H., Schmid-Burgk, W., Holzmuller, B. (1980). Low cerebrospinal fluid glutamate in schizophrenic patients and a new hypothesis on schizophrenia. *Neurosci Lett*, 20, 379–82.

Krystal, J. H., Karper, L. P., Seibyl, J. P., et al. (1994). Subanesthetic effects of the noncompetitive NMDA antagonist, ketamine, in humans. Psychotomimetic, perceptual, cognitive, and neuroendocrine responses. *Arch Gen Psychiatry*, 51, 199–214.

Lahti, A. C., Koffel, B., Laporte, D., Tamminga, C. A. (1995). Subanesthetic doses of ketamine stimulate psychosis in schizophrenia. *Neuropsychopharmacology*, 13, 9–19.

Loebel, A., Cucchiaro, J., Sarma, K., et al. (2013). Efficacy and safety of lurasidone 80 mg/day and 160 mg/day in the treatment of schizophrenia: a randomized, double-blind, placebo- and active-controlled trial. *Schizophr Res*, 145, 101–9.

Loebel, A., Silva, R., Goldman, R., et al. (2016). Lurasidone dose escalation in early nonresponding patients with schizophrenia: a randomized, placebo-controlled study. *J Clin Psychiatry*, 77, 1672–80.

Meltzer, H. Y. (1989). Clinical studies on the mechanism of action of clozapine: the dopamine-serotonin hypothesis of schizophrenia. *Psychopharmacology (Berl)*, 99 (Suppl), S18–27.

Meltzer, H. Y., Elkis, H., Vanover, K., et al. (2012). Pimavanserin, a selective serotonin (5-HT)2A-inverse agonist, enhances the efficacy and safety of risperidone, 2mg/day, but does not enhance efficacy of haloperidol, 2mg/day: comparison with reference dose risperidone, 6mg/day. *Schizophr Res*, 141, 144–52.

Merritt, K., Egerton, A., Kempton, M. J., Taylor, M. J., McGuire, P. K. (2016). Nature of glutamate alterations in schizophrenia: a meta-analysis of proton magnetic resonance spectroscopy studies. *JAMA Psychiatry*, 73, 665–74.

Mouchlianitis, E., Bloomfield, M. A., Law, V., et al. (2016). Treatment-resistant schizophrenia patients show elevated anterior cingulate cortex glutamate compared to treatment-responsive. *Schizophr Bull*, 42, 744–52.

Nordstrom, A. L., Farde, L., Nyberg, S., Karlsson, P., Halldin, C., Sedvall, G. (1995). D1, D2, and 5-HT2 receptor occupancy in relation to clozapine serum concentration: a PET study of schizophrenic patients. *Am J Psychiatry*, 152, 1444–9.

Nyberg, S., Farde, L., Halldin, C., Dahl, M. L., Bertilsson, L. (1995). D2 dopamine receptor occupancy during low-dose treatment with haloperidol decanoate. *Am J Psychiatry*, 152, 173–8.

Ottong, S. E., Garver, D. L. (1997). A biomodal distribution of plasma HVA/MHPG in the psychoses. *Psychiatry Res,* 69, 97–103.

Pilowsky, L. S., Costa, D. C., Ell, P. J., Murray, R. M., Verhoeff, N. P., Kerwin, R. W. (1993). Antipsychotic medication, D2 dopamine receptor blockade and clinical response: a 123I IBZM SPET (single photon emission tomography) study. *Psychol Med,* 23, 791–7.

Potkin, S. G., Basile, V. S., Jin, Y., et al. (2003). D1 receptor alleles predict PET metabolic correlates of clinical response to clozapine. *Mol Psychiatry,* 8, 109–13.

Potkin, S. G., Keator, D. B., Kesler-West, M. L., et al. (2014). D2 receptor occupancy following lurasidone treatment in patients with schizophrenia or schizoaffective disorder. *CNS Spectrums,* 19, 176–81.

Remington, G., Kapur, S. (2010). Antipsychotic dosing: how much but also how often? *Schizophr Bull,* 36, 900–3.

Richtand, N. M., Welge, J. A., Logue, A. D., et al. (2007). Dopamine and serotonin receptor binding and antipsychotic efficacy. *Neuropsychopharmacology,* 32, 1715.

Roberts, R. C., Roche, J. K., Conley, R. R., Lahti, A. C. (2009). Dopaminergic synapses in the caudate of subjects with schizophrenia: relationship to treatment response. *Synapse (New York, N.Y.),* 63, 520–30.

Ross, S. B., Renyi, A. L. (1967). Inhibition of the uptake of tritiated catecholamines by antidepressant and related agents. *Eur J Pharmacol,* 2, 181–6.

Rothman, D. L., Behar, K. L., Hyder, F., Shulman, R. G. (2003). In vivo NMR studies of the glutamate neurotransmitter flux and neuroenergetics: implications for brain function. *Annu Rev Physiol,* 65, 401–27.

Samaha, A.-N., Seeman, P., Stewart, J., Rajabi, H., Kapur, S. (2007). 'Breakthrough' dopamine supersensitivity during ongoing antipsychotic treatment leads to treatment failure over time. *J Neurosci,* 27, 2979–86.

Seeman, P. (2001). Antipsychotic drugs, dopamine receptors, and schizophrenia. *Clin Neurosci Res,* 1, 53–60.

Seeman, P. (2013). Schizophrenia and dopamine receptors. *Eur Neuropsychopharmacol,* 23, 999–1009.

Seeman, P., Lee, T. (1975). Antipsychotic drugs: direct correlation between clinical potency and presynaptic action on dopamine neurons. *Science,* 188, 1217–19.

Seeman, P., Chau-Wong, M., Tedesco, J., Wong, K. (1975). Brain receptors for antipsychotic drugs and dopamine: direct binding assays. *Proc Natl Acad Sci USA,* 72, 4376–80.

Seeman, P., Lee, T., Chau-Wong, M., Wong, K. (1976). Antipsychotic drug doses and neuroleptic/dopamine receptors. *Nature,* 261, 717–19.

Seeman, P., Bzowej, N. H., Guan, H. C., et al. (1987). Human brain D1 and D2 dopamine receptors in schizophrenia, Alzheimer's, Parkinson's, and Huntington's diseases. *Neuropsychopharmacology,* 1, 5–15.

Selvaraj, S., Arnone, D., Cappai, A., Howes, O. (2014). Alterations in the serotonin system in schizophrenia: a systematic review and meta-analysis of postmortem and molecular imaging studies. *Neurosci Biobehav Rev,* 45, 233–45.

Silvestri, S., Seeman, M. V., Negrete, J. C., et al. (2000). Increased dopamine D2 receptor binding after long-term treatment with antipsychotics in humans: a clinical PET study. *Psychopharmacology (Berl),* 152, 174–80.

CHAPTER 5

Spano, P. F., Govoni, S., Trabucchi, M. (1978). Studies on the pharmacological properties of dopamine receptors in various areas of the central nervous system. *Adv Biochem Psychopharmacol,* 19, 155–65.

Stone, J. M., Morrison, P. D., Pilowsky, L. S. (2007). Glutamate and dopamine dysregulation in schizophrenia—a synthesis and selective review. *J Psychopharmacol,* 21, 440–52.

Thompson, J. L., Urban, N., Slifstein, M., et al. (2013). Striatal dopamine release in schizophrenia comorbid with substance dependence. *Mol Psychiatry,* 18, 909–15.

Wolkin, A., Barouche, F., Wolf, A. P., et al. (1989). Dopamine blockade and clinical response: evidence for two biological subgroups of schizophrenia. *Am J Psychiatry,* 146, 905–8.

Yoshimura, R., Ueda, N., Shinkai, K., Nakamura, J. (2003). Plasma levels of homovanillic acid and the response to risperidone in first episode untreated acute schizophrenia. *Int Clin Psychopharmacol,* 18, 107–11.

Zumárraga, M., González-Torres, M. A., Arrue, A., et al. (2011). Variability of plasma homovanillic acid over 13 months in patients with schizophrenia; relationship with the clinical response and the Wisconsin card sort test. *Neurochemical Res,* 36, 1336–43.

CHAPTER 5

Pharmacological management of treatment-resistant schizophrenia: fundamentals of clozapine

Yvonne Yang and Stephen Marder

KEY POINTS

- Evidence from controlled clinical trials supports the prescribing of clozapine for patients with treatment-resistant schizophrenia (TRS).

- Early studies focused on severely ill TRS patients. More recent studies indicate that clozapine can also be effective for patients who are relatively stable but are burdened by persistent psychotic symptoms.

- Clozapine treatment is associated with a substantial side effect burden, including sedation, orthostasis, weight gain, constipation, and seizures. In addition, because of a risk of potentially fatal agranulocytosis, clozapine patients require regular monitoring of their neutrophil count.

- Measuring clozapine plasma concentrations can be helpful in managing patients with severe side effects and those with an inadequate clinical response.

- A trial of clozapine should consist of a minimum duration of 12 weeks.

Effectiveness of clozapine in treatment-resistant schizophrenia

When clozapine was first evaluated as an antipsychotic, it was notable for being an effective antipsychotic with negligible extrapyramidal side effects (EPS). However, deaths from agranulocytosis and subsequent infections led to the withdrawal of clozapine in European countries where it had been approved. Attempts to withdraw clozapine in some patients led to the observation that other antipsychotics could not duplicate clozapine's therapeutic effects. Moreover, regular monitoring of white blood cell counts in these individuals showed that clozapine-induced agranulocytosis was reversible if clozapine was discontinued. With this safety monitoring, clinicians in Europe and the USA were permitted to prescribe clozapine to selected severely ill patients for humanitarian reasons. The reported effectiveness of clozapine in these individuals led to studies evaluating whether clozapine was effective for patients who failed to respond to available antipsychotics.

Controlled trials in Europe (Fischer-Cornelssen and Ferner, 1976) found that clozapine's advantage over chlorpromazine was most obvious in the most severely ill schizophrenia patients. This study, along with clinical experience, led to a multicentre trial comparing clozapine and chlorpromazine in patients who had a history of poor response to antipsychotics based both on their treatment history and a prospective trial of haloperidol (Kane et al., 1988). In this 6-week trial, the clozapine-treated patients did better on a range of measures of both positive and negative symptoms relative to chlorpromazine. Thirty per cent of clozapine-treated patients met a priori criteria for significant improvement, in contrast to only 4% of chlorpromazine-treated patients. There is also evidence that the proportion of patients meeting improvement criteria would have been higher if the trial had been longer than 6 weeks (Kane et al., 2001).

More recent studies indicate that clozapine also has advantages for TRS patients who are less severely ill and able to live in their communities. The National Institute of Mental Health (NIMH) Clinical Antipsychotic Trials of Intervention Effectiveness (CATIE) compared clozapine with risperidone, olanzapine, or quetiapine in outpatients with schizophrenia who had failed to show response in an earlier phase of the study because of a lack of efficacy (McEvoy et al., 2006). Patients treated with clozapine had the lowest discontinuation rates, with 56% of patients on clozapine discontinuing treatment, compared with 71% of those on olanzapine, 86% of those on risperidone, and 93% of those on quetiapine. A trial from the UK, the Cost Utility of the Latest Antipsychotic Drugs in Schizophrenia Study—band 2 (CUtLASS-2) (Lewis et al., 2006), assigned outpatients who had responded poorly to two prior antipsychotics to either clozapine or a second-generation antipsychotic (SGA) selected prior to randomization. Patients who received clozapine demonstrated greater improvement than those on the comparison drugs. Other trials with subjects who are defined as having only moderate persistent symptoms also support clozapine's effectiveness (Kane et al., 2001; Schooler et al., 2016).

Most meta-analyses of clinical trials have supported clozapine's advantages. For example, a meta-analysis (Leucht et al., 2013) of commonly prescribed antipsychotic medications used both direct and indirect comparisons and found that clozapine was the most effective antipsychotic. A meta-analysis of head-to-head comparisons of clozapine to first-generation antipsychotics (FGAs) and SGAs also found that clozapine was superior for positive symptoms in both short- and long-term trials (Siskind et al., 2016). In contrast, a network meta-analysis (Samara et al., 2016) failed to find an advantage of clozapine in TRS. However, this meta-analysis used a methodology that may have underestimated clozapine's efficacy (Kane and Correll, 2016).

In summary, there is compelling evidence that clozapine is the most effective medication for TRS. It supports the guideline from the Schizophrenia Patient Outcome Research Team that clozapine should be offered to patients who have 'persistent and clinically significant' positive symptoms despite treatment with two antipsychotic medications (Buchanan et al., 2010).

Assessing patients for clozapine

Before starting a patient on clozapine, the clinician should ensure that the patient has an absolute neutrophil count (ANC) of at least 1500/μL for the general population and 1000/μL if the individual has a documented history of benign ethnic neutropenia (BEN). We also recommend a baseline electrocardiogram before starting clozapine. Since clozapine can be associated with weight gain and the development of insulin resistance, we also recommend ordering a baseline fasting blood glucose or haemoglobin A1c and a lipid panel.

Contraindications

There are no absolute contraindications against the use of clozapine, with the exception of a known hypersensitivity reaction to clozapine (Clozapine REMS Patient Safety Information). Caution should be used in patients with known seizure disorders, glaucoma, prostatic enlargement, significant cardiac disease, obesity, or diabetes. For instance, patients with seizure disorders ideally should be stabilized on antiepileptic medication prior to initiation of clozapine. Patients with obesity or diabetes should undergo standard monitoring while on clozapine. However, even patients who have experienced potentially fatal side effects such as agranulocytosis or myocarditis from clozapine may be re-challenged carefully. The risk versus benefit of clozapine should be considered for each patient on a case-by-case basis.

Initiation and titration

In the USA, to initiate clozapine treatment, the prescriber, pharmacy, and patient must be enrolled in the Clozapine Risk Evaluation and Mitigation Strategy (REMS) program (www.clozapinerems.com); similar monitoring schemes exist in many other countries. A baseline absolute neutrophil count (ANC) must be obtained via standard complete blood count (CBC) with differential. Baseline ANC must be at least 1500/μL for the general population or 1000/μL for patients with BEN for initiation of clozapine treatment. CBC must then be monitored weekly for 6 months, every 2 weeks for the subsequent 6 months, and every 4 weeks thereafter, for the duration of clozapine treatment, or the pharmacy will be unable to dispense the medication to the patient.

Benign ethnic neutropenia

Approximately 10–30% of patients of African, Arabian, or Mediterranean descent will present with BEN (Manu et al., 2016). This condition, thought to have evolved in response to the existence of malaria in these geographical regions, results in an approximate 500/μL to 800/μL reduction in baseline neutrophils with no resultant effect on immune performance. Patients with BEN diagnosed by a haematologist may initiate clozapine treatment with a baseline ANC of 1000/μL or greater.

Titration schedules

In the outpatient setting, clozapine should be started at low doses and increased slowly to minimize side effect burden, reduce risk of agranulocytosis and other adverse reactions, and increase likelihood of patient adherence. The starting dose should be 12.5–25 mg per os daily and be divided into twice-a-day dosing initially. Rates of titration vary depending on numerous factors, including feasibility of frequent visits on the part of the patient or provider, side effect burden (usually somnolence) experienced by the patient, and cognitive burden of a complicated titration schedule.

A relatively rapid example titration schedule from the clozapine manufacturer Teva is outlined in Table 6.1. It achieves a 300-mg dose at the end of 2 weeks (Teva Pharmaceuticals, 2017).

Subsequent increases may be made at a maximum of 100 mg/week, as tolerated by the patient. The maximum dose of clozapine per day recommended by the Clozapine REMS Program is 900 mg/day. On an inpatient unit, a slightly faster titration schedule may be utilized in light of more frequent monitoring for side effects and potentially life-threatening adverse reactions. Conversely, in the outpatient setting, a slower titration should be used for patients who may experience difficulty with complicated titration regimens. A slower regimen may also allow patients more time to accommodate to side effects such as sedation, which can be severe even at very low doses.

Dose and dosing regimen

The initial target dose for titration is 300–450 mg/day (Novartis Pharmaceuticals, 2015); however, in our experience, patients can do well on substantially lower doses. With a mean half-life of 12 hours after reaching steady-state on a 100-mg

Table 6.1 Example clozapine titration schedule from the manufacturer Teva

Week 1	am dose (mg)	pm dose (mg)	Total daily dose (mg)	Week 2	am dose (mg)	pm dose (mg)	Total daily dose (mg)
Day 1	12.5	12.5 (optional)	12.5–25	Day 8	75	100	175
Day 2	25	—	25	Day 9	100	100	200
Day 3	25	25	50	Day 10	100	125	225
Day 4	25	50	75	Day 11	100	150	250
Day 5	50	50	100	Day 12	125	150	275
Day 6	50	75	125	Day 13	150	150	300
Day 7	50	100	150	Day 14	150	150	300

twice-daily clozapine dose, patients may benefit from twice-daily dosing; however, most patients do well with once a day dosing in the evening. Twice-daily dosing may be utilized to ameliorate side effects or for patients with persistent morning psychosis or agitation.

Drug–drug interactions that should be taken into consideration when prescribing clozapine include inducers and inhibitors of the cytochrome P450 enzymes CYP1A2, CYP2D6, and CYP3A4. Moderate CYP3A4 inducers such as cigarette smoke and carbamazepine, phenytoin, St. John's wort, and rifampicin reduce clozapine levels. Therefore, smoking patients and patients on these medications may require higher doses of clozapine. Caution should be used upon discontinuation of these medications or with smoking cessation, as patients may require a reduction in clozapine dose.

When coadministered with strong CYP1A2 inhibitors (e.g. fluvoxamine or the fluoroquinolones ciprofloxacin and enoxacin), the clozapine dose should be reduced by one-third. Other CYP1A2, CYP2D6, and CYP3A4 inhibitors can also increase clozapine doses, and dose reduction should be considered in these cases (e.g. oral contraceptives, caffeine, cimetidine, escitalopram, erythromycin, paroxetine, bupropion, fluoxetine, quinidine, duloxetine, terbinafine, sertraline).

Physical health monitoring

Absolute neutrophil count monitoring

ANC must be monitored carefully for reductions that could signal agranulocytosis. Please see package insert for detailed monitoring guidelines (Novartis Pharmaceuticals, 2015; Teva Pharmaceuticals, 2017). In general, an ANC of 1000/μL to 1499/μL is regarded as mild neutropenia, ANC 500/μL to 999/μL as moderate neutropenia, and ANC <500/μL as severe neutropenia. In the case of mild neutropenia, clozapine treatment may continue with more frequent monitoring (three times weekly blood draws until ANC normalizes). If moderate or severe neutropenia occur, clozapine treatment must be interrupted, and a haematology consultation is recommended. For patients with BEN, a drop in ANC is defined as neutropenia if ANC is 500/μL to 999/μL, and severe neutropenia if ANC <500/μL. Clozapine should be interrupted in BEN patients with severe neutropenia.

Side effect monitoring

Patients on clozapine are susceptible to weight gain and insulin resistance and require regular health monitoring to prevent development of these adverse effects. Consensus guidelines were developed by the American Diabetes Association in 2004 and continue to be the main guide in the USA for health monitoring (American Diabetes Association et al., 2004). Their findings are reproduced in Table 6.2.

Table 6.2 Consensus guidelines for health monitoring to prevent diabetes and obesity

Risk factor	Timing of assessment					
	First year of antipsychotic				Ongoing monitoring*	
	Baseline	6 weeks	3 months	12 months	Quarterly[¶]	Annually[¶]
Personal and family history of diabetes, hypertension, or cardiovascular disease	X					X
Smoking status, physical activity, diet[Δ]	X	X	X		X	
Weight, body mass index[Δ]	X	X	X		X	
Blood pressure[Δ]	X	X	X		X	
Fasting glucose or HbA1c[◊]	X	X[§]	X	X		X
Lipid profile (fasting or non-fasting)	X		X	X		X

* In subsequent years of antipsychotic and in patients with severe mental illness.

[¶] Ongoing quarterly and annual monitoring is appropriate when health indicators are within the normal range. More frequent monitoring is indicated when health indicators are out of range.

[Δ] Assess regularly as part of general health maintenance.

[◊] HbA1c is usually more practical to obtain than fasting glucose but either can be used.

[§] Fasting glucose at six weeks is only recommended by European guidelines, but given evidence for rapid-onset hyperglycemia in some individuals starting antipsychotics, this represents prudent monitoring, especially for clozapine and olanzapine.

Reproduced with permission from: Marder S, Stroup S. Pharmacotherapy for schizophrenia: Side effect management. In: UpToDate, Post TW (Ed), UpToDate, Waltham, MA. (Accessed on 24.7.2018.) Copyright © 2018 UpToDate, Inc. For more information visit www.uptodate.com.

Source data from *Nature Reviews Endocrinology*, 8, De Hert M, Detraux J, van Winkel R, et al., Metabolic and cardiovascular adverse effects associated with antipsychotic drugs, 2011

Use of clozapine plasma levels

Measuring clozapine plasma concentrations may be useful in managing many patients. A number of studies (e.g. Potkin et al., 1994; Miller, 1996) have found that patients who have concentrations in the range of 350–400 ng/mL are more likely to respond than those with lower concentrations. Higher levels, such as 600 ng/mL or higher, do not appear to be more effective and are probably associated with more severe side effects, including a risk of seizures. If the laboratory is reporting both the parent drug and norclozapine, levels will be higher.

We do not recommend the routine monitoring of plasma concentrations. However, plasma levels may be helpful in certain circumstances. For example, if patients are experiencing side effects, and responding well to clozapine, plasma levels may encourage reducing the dose. Alternatively, if patients are not responding well, a low plasma level will support increasing the dose.

The duration of clozapine trials

Given the side effect burden of a clozapine trial, patients and family members may pressure clinicians to discontinue clozapine within the first weeks of treatment. Since it may take several weeks for patients to achieve an optimal clozapine dose, a trial of this medication is likely to be longer than a trial with other antipsychotics. An early study (Conley et al., 1997) found that the mean time to response for patients with TRS was about 82 days, although patients may have responded sooner. The study also found that patients responded within 8 weeks of a dosage increase. This suggests that patients should receive a trial which is at least 3 months. If there is some evidence of improvement after 3 months we recommend that patients receive clozapine for an additional 3 months before determining whether response is adequate.

REFERENCES

American Diabetes Association, American Psychiatric Association, American Association of Clinical Endocrinologists, North American Association for the Study of Obesity (2004). Consensus Development Conference on Antipsychotic Drugs and Obesity and Diabetes. *Diabetes Care*, 27(2), 596–601.

Buchanan, R. W., Kreyenbuhl, J., Kelly, D. L. et al., Schizophrenia Patient Outcomes Research (2010). The 2009 schizophrenia PORT psychopharmacological treatment recommendations and summary statements. *Schizophr Bull*, 36(1), 71–93.

Conley, R. R., Carpenter, W. T. Jr., Tamminga, C. A. (1997). Time to clozapine response in a standardized trial. *Am J Psychiatry*, 154(9), 1243–7.

Fischer-Cornelssen, K. A., Ferner, U. J. (1976). An example of European multicenter trials: multispectral analysis of clozapine. *Psychopharmacol Bull*, 12(2), 34–9.

Kane, J. M., Correll, C. U. (2016). The role of clozapine in treatment-resistant schizophrenia. *JAMA Psychiatry*, 73(3), 187–8.

Kane, J., Honigfeld, G., Singer, J., Meltzer, H. (1988). Clozapine for the treatment-resistant schizophrenic. A double-blind comparison with chlorpromazine. *Arch Gen Psychiatry,* 45(9), 789–96.

Kane, J. M., Marder, S. R., Schooler, N. R. et al. (2001). Clozapine and haloperidol in moderately refractory schizophrenia: a 6-month randomized and double-blind comparison. *Arch Gen Psychiatry,* 58(10), 965–72.

Leucht, S., Cipriani, A., Spineli, L. et al. (2013). Comparative efficacy and tolerability of 15 antipsychotic drugs in schizophrenia: a multiple-treatments meta-analysis. *Lancet,* 382(9896), 951–62.

Lewis, S. W., Barnes, T. R., Davies, L., et al. (2006). Randomized controlled trial of effect of prescription of clozapine versus other second-generation antipsychotic drugs in resistant schizophrenia. *Schizophr Bull,* 32(4), 715–23.

Manu, P., Sarvaiya, N., Rogozea, L. M., Kane, J. M., Correll, C. U. (2016). Benign ethnic neutropenia and clozapine use: a systematic review of the evidence and treatment recommendations. *J Clin Psychiatry,* 77(7), e909–16.

McEvoy, J. P., Lieberman, J. A., Stroup, T. S. et al. and CATIE Investigators (2006). Effectiveness of clozapine versus olanzapine, quetiapine, and risperidone in patients with chronic schizophrenia who did not respond to prior atypical antipsychotic treatment. *Am J Psychiatry,* 163(4), 600–10.

Miller, D. D. (1996). The clinical use of clozapine plasma concentrations in the management of treatment-refractory schizophrenia. *Ann Clin Psychiatry,* 8(2), 99–109.

Novartis Pharmaceuticals. (2015). CLOZARIL Prescribing Information. Available at: http://clozaril.com/wp-content/themes/eyesite/pi/Clozaril_PI.pdf [Accessed 24 October, 2017].

Potkin, S. G., Bera, R., Gulasekaram, B., et al. (1994). Plasma clozapine concentrations predict clinical response in treatment-resistant schizophrenia. *J Clin Psychiatry,* 55 (Suppl. B), 133–6.

Samara, M. T., Dold, M., Gianatsi, M., et al. (2016). Efficacy, acceptability, and tolerability of antipsychotics in treatment-resistant schizophrenia: a network meta-analysis. *JAMA Psychiatry,* 73(3), 199–210.

Schooler, N. R., Marder, S. R., Chengappa, K. N., et al. (2016). Clozapine and risperidone in moderately refractory schizophrenia: a 6-month randomized double-blind comparison. *J Clin Psychiatry,* 77(5), 628–34.

Siskind, D., McCartney, L., Goldschlager, R., Kisely, S. (2016). Clozapine v. first- and second-generation antipsychotics in treatment-refractory schizophrenia: systematic review and meta-analysis. *Br J Psychiatry,* 209(5), 385–92.

Teva Pharmaceuticals. (2017). Teva example clozapine titration. Available at: http://tevaclozapine.com/documents/TitrationSalesAid_10601_Final.pdf [Accessed 24 October, 2017].

CHAPTER 7

Managing common adverse effects of clozapine

Christopher Rohde and Jimmi Nielsen

KEY POINTS

- Adverse effects during clozapine treatment are common, and can be divided into very common (>10%: constipation, weight gain, metabolic side effects, sedation, and sialorrhea), common (1–10%: seizures and enuresis), and cardiac (sinus tachycardia, electrocardiogram [ECG] abnormalities, and orthostatic hypotension) adverse effects.

- Most adverse effects are benign, but they may often reduce the quality of life for the patient, leading to reduced adherence and thereby psychotic relapse.

- Treatment of these adverse effects is important and should not be neglected. In this chapter, we present specific treatment strategies for each adverse effect.

- Most side effects of clozapine can be effectively treated, but this requires being proactive.

- This chapter presents specific treatment strategies for common adverse effects of clozapine.

Introduction

The effect of clozapine in treatment-resistant schizophrenia has been documented in several studies (Kane et al., 1988; McEvoy et al., 2006; Nielsen et al., 2012). Despite lack of response to previous treatment, up to two-thirds of these patients may respond to clozapine (Nielsen et al., 2012). Treating patients with clozapine is complicated by the complex pharmacokinetic and pharmacodynamic properties of clozapine and the ability of clozapine to cause several idiosyncratic adverse effects. Although the receptor profile of clozapine is well known, the exact unique therapeutic mechanism remains largely unknown and cannot solely be attributed to a single receptor. In contrast, the most common adverse effects can often be explained to the affinity of one or more receptors.

The aim of this chapter is to illustrate the management of the most common adverse effects of clozapine, first by covering the general managing strategies of clozapine and then by describing the management of the specific adverse effects. Unfortunately, it is beyond the scope of this chapter to cover the management of the rare idiosyncratic adverse effects, and psychiatrists are recommended to search the relevant literature elsewhere (Nielsen et al., 2013). As most patients treated with clozapine are non-responders to other antipsychotics, there is a need for psychiatrists to have substantial knowledge on how to manage the most common adverse effects of clozapine to maintain the patient on clozapine.

General management strategies

Most of the common adverse effects are type A adverse effects (mnemonic: augmented) and show dose dependency, at least to some degree (Edwards and Aronson, 2000). This emphasizes the importance of treating patients with the lowest effective dose, i.e. the benefits of the last 100 mg are often only minor compared to the increasing burden of adverse effects. As a consequence, dose reduction should always be considered if possible, but may not be possible owing to the risk of psychotic relapse. Although dosing should be based on clinical effects and adverse effects, therapeutic drug monitoring may assist in finding the optimum dose.

Usually doses are divided into several doses, often with the highest dose at bedtime. A single bedtime dose can be used for up to 400–500 mg/day, but it is often necessary to divide into two or more doses at higher dosages. Many adverse effects can be managed by simply changing the distribution of doses, e.g. instead of adding a benzodiazepine for comorbid anxiety, a smaller dose of the total clozapine dose during the day may alleviate this problem and reduce the burden of side effects. Although the evidence for use of clozapine-sparing antipsychotics is not solid, it may still be a useful strategy to reduce the burden of side effects. At a receptor level point of view, the clozapine-sparing drug should have minimal affinity for histamine or noradrenergic alpha-1 receptors as these are usually dose-limiting factors with clozapine. Another option to address clozapine-associated adverse effects is to start specific rescue medication, as described in Fig. 7.1.

Very common (>10%) adverse effects

Constipation

Constipation is one of the most common adverse effects during clozapine treatment; up to one-third of patients will develop constipation at some point, with

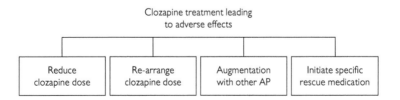

Fig. 7.1 General managing strategies. AP, Antipsychotic.

the highest risk within the first 4 months (Shirazi et al., 2016). Clozapine-induced constipation is mainly caused by the anticholinergic effect of clozapine, but also antagonism of histamine receptors may contribute because of sedation and reduced physical activity (Shirazi et al., 2016).

Management of constipation is important as, in severe cases, it may be fatal due to ileus, perforation, and gastrointestinal ischaemia. In addition, patients with schizophrenia and other serious mental disorders rarely complain about abdominal pain owing to altered pain sensitivity (Palmer et al., 2008), which increases the risk of more severe complications as diagnosis is often delayed.

As constipation occurs with other antipsychotic drugs, screening of bowel habits before clozapine is initiated is recommended. If defaecation frequency is lower than 4–5 times per week, treatment is warranted before clozapine is initiated. Screening of bowel habits should be performed at least bi-weekly during the first 3 months and then quarterly.

Although non-pharmacological intervention, such as exercise, fluid, and fibre intake, may not be sufficient and its use is complicated by low compliance, it is highly recommended. The evidence for pharmacological treatment of clozapine-induced constipation remains sparse (Every-Palmer et al., 2017). However, traditionally used pharmacological agents for constipation, such as osmotic laxatives, bulk-forming laxatives, stool softeners, and stimulant laxatives (Costilla and Foxx-Orenstein, 2014), should be initiated, even in combination, to achieve defaecation at least 4–5 times per week as this prevents the development of ileus (Shirazi et al., 2016) (Table 7.1). In addition, other drugs associated with constipation, such as opioids and anticholinergic drugs, should be tapered off if possible and prescribed with caution (Bishara and Taylor, 2014).

In our practice, the best way to manage patients developing constipation is to initiate non-pharmacological treatment together with lactulose or magnesium oxide when the first signs of constipation develop. These products are cheap and can easily be purchased, which is likely to increase compliance. For most patients, this combination is sufficient and will lead to normal defaecation patterns. Patients should be encouraged to drink plenty of water as fluid is necessary with these laxatives. If the stool frequency does not improve within 2 weeks, we recommend adding a stimulant laxative for a short period of time. Long-term use of stimulant laxatives is rarely warranted.

Weight gain and metabolic side effects

Treatment with clozapine is often associated with substantial weight gain and metabolic side effects, i.e. abdominal obesity, arterial hypertension, elevated blood glucose, low high-density lipoprotein cholesterol, and hypertriglyceridaemia (De Hert et al., 2011). As a result, body weight, body mass index (BMI), waist circumference, blood pressure, HbA1c, and lipids should be monitored closely after clozapine initiation and then yearly, as it is important to recognize these harmful conditions early so that relevant interventions can be initiated.

Table 7.1 Management of very common adverse effects of clozapine

Type	Management strategy	Discontinuation	Clinical comments
Constipation	Treatment should be initiated if frequency of defaecation is lower than 4–5 times per week. *Non-pharmacological intervention*: Exercise, fluid, and fibre intake. *Pharmacological intervention*: Bulk-forming laxatives, stool softeners, osmotic laxatives (lactulose, magnesium oxide, or polyethylene glycol), stimulant laxatives (bisacodyl or sodium picosulfate).	Rare reason for discontinuation, but ileus or subileus should lead to pause.	Compliance of non-pharmacological interventions is often low and treatment effect not sufficient. In such cases, start with osmotic laxatives and only use stimulant laxatives in case of non-response.
Weight gain	Weight should be monitored closely after clozapine initiation. *Non-pharmacological intervention*: Early behavioural interventions, including diet modification and nutritional counselling. *Pharmacological intervention*: Aripiprazole, fluvoxamine, topiramate, GLP-1 receptor antagonist, or metformin.	No reason for discontinuation.	In case non-pharmacological interventions are not sufficient, we recommend use of aripiprazole as first-line treatment. Despite, several pharmacological interventions available, weight remains a major issue.
Metabolic syndrome	Waist circumference, blood pressure, HbA1c, and lipids should be monitored closely after clozapine initiation. Treatment should follow common medical guidelines. Metabolic side effects are associated with weight gain and can be minimized by reducing the weight gain.	No reason for discontinuation.	

continued >

Table 7.1 Management of very common adverse effects of clozapine *(continued)*

Type	Management strategy	Discontinuation	Clinical comments
Sedation	Likely to diminish after 4–6 weeks of treatment. Use minimum effective dose, slow up-titration, and giving the majority at night may be helpful. Augmentation with aripiprazole should be considered.	No reason for discontinuation.	Use of central nervous system stimulants is not recommended owing to risk of psychotic relapse.
Sialorrhea	Likely to diminish after 4–6 weeks of treatment. Use minimum effective dose and apply largest dose at nighttime. *Non-pharmacological interventions*: Chewing gum during daytime and elevated position while sleeping. *Pharmacological interventions*: Anticholinergic drugs (biperiden). α_2-antiadrenergic drugs (clonidine). Atropine drops sublingually. Other possibilities include amisulpride, sulpiride, and moclobemide.	No reason for discontinuation.	Most patients accept nighttime drooling and focus should be to alleviate daytime drooling. Although, atropine drops are usually effective, clozapine-sparing antipsychotics may be necessary.

If the patient starts gaining weight, early healthy lifestyle guidance is important to prevent an uncontrolled weight gain. Combined behavioural interventions, consisting of both diet modification and nutritional counselling, are effective (Whitney et al., 2015), preferably in combination with exercise (Wu et al., 2007). If non-pharmacological treatment is insufficient, some pharmacological drugs have been suggested (Whitney et al., 2015). Aripiprazole (at 5–10 mg/day) in combination with clozapine has been shown to decrease body weight and reduce BMI (Henderson et al., 2006). However, keep in mind the risk that the combination of antipsychotic drugs may increase the risk of other adverse effects. Fluvoxamine has in one study been suggested to attenuate clozapine-induced weight gain (Lu et al., 2004), but it is recommended that plasma concentration of clozapine is monitored if these drugs are combined, as fluvoxamine inhibits the metabolism of clozapine. Topiramate (Afshar et al., 2009; Hahn et al., 2010) and metformin (Carrizo et al., 2009; Chen et al., 2013) have also been shown to induce weight gain in patients treated with clozapine. Recently, GLP-1 antagonists have shown promising effects in clozapine-induced weight gain (Larsen et al., 2017). However, it is important to emphasize that non-pharmacological treatment is the first choice for preventing weight gain.

Hyperglycaemia, hypertension, and dyslipidaemia should be treated according to common medical guidelines, including metformin, angiotensin-converting enzyme (ACE) inhibitors, and statins. The metabolic side effects can be prevented by using the same strategies previously mentioned, as they are often associated with weight gain.

Neither weight gain nor metabolic side effects should be reasons for discontinuation of clozapine. Although some dose dependency has been found with clozapine-induced weight gain (de Leon et al., 2007), dose reduction is seldom enough to reduce or reverse weight gain.

We propose the following steps when a patient starts gaining weight after clozapine initiation. First, we recommend a consultation with the doctor and a dietitian to identify how lifestyle can be improved to reduce weight gain. Many calories are often spent on sugar-containing beverages and it may be effective to reduce intake of soda and coffee with sugar. Another focus is to reduce the amount of fast food and instead introduce a more regular eating pattern as this may reduce the total intake of calories.

Professionals should focus both on healthier eating habits but also on how to change sedentary lifestyle and on initiating regular exercise. If weight gain continues, we recommend adding aripiprazole and, if possible, reduce the dose of clozapine. Metformin should be reserved for those with glucose intolerance.

Sedation

The histaminergic antagonistic effect of clozapine is considered to be responsible for sedation, which is a very common adverse effect of clozapine treatment. The clozapine-associated sedation will often diminish after 4–6 weeks of treatment, as tachyphylaxis occurs (Young et al., 1998). Informing the patient about the sedative effect and that it is likely to diminish after a few weeks is often enough for the patient to endure this adverse effect. In addition, using the minimum effective dose, slow up-titration, and giving the major portion at night are usually beneficial. Augmentation with aripiprazole or another non-sedating antipsychotic may be helpful in severe cases, but further research is warranted (Perdigues et al., 2016).

In our experience, most patients accept the sedation if they are informed that it will diminish after 4–6 weeks. To diminish sedation, we give all or the largest dose of clozapine at nighttime. With doses higher than 400–500 mg we give the rest in the morning and/or during the day, guided by patient preference. Only in cases of persisting sedation do we recommend adding a clozapine-sparing drug, e.g. aripiprazole, and subsequently reducing the dose of clozapine. Remember also to taper off other sedating drugs, such as mirtazapine, antihistamines, or benzodiazepines, if possible.

Although case reports have suggested use of central nervous system stimulants for clozapine-induced sedation, we do not recommend this as, in theory, it may increase the risk of psychotic relapse (Rohde et al., 2017).

Sialorrhea (hypersalivation)

Hypersalivation is a common side effect to clozapine, occurring in 30–80% of patients (Miller, 2000). The mechanism for paradoxical clozapine-induced hypersalivation remains largely unclear, as its anticholinergic effect should provide the opposite effect. Hypersalivation may lead to drooling at night, and both symptoms can be very debilitating for the patient, leading to skin damage around the mouth with secondary infection, sleeping difficulties, choking sensation, aspiration, pneumonia, chronic cough, and stigmatization (Sagy et al., 2014; Praharaj et al., 2006). As these complications can very well lead to discontinuation of clozapine, it is important to initiate pharmacological and non-pharmacological treatment strategies if the symptom develops.

Non-pharmacological treatment during daytime includes chewing gum to promote swallowing and, for night-time, elevating the head position using extra pillows while sleeping. Patients with risk of aspiration can be encouraged to sleep in the lateral decubitus position. Pharmacological treatment includes numerous different medications (Sagy et al., 2014). The first step is to find the minimum effective dose of clozapine, as this side effect is largely dose-dependent. If the hypersalivation continues, anticholinergic medication or an alpha-2-adrenoreceptor agonist, such as biperiden and clonidine, respectively, can be administered, but with the risk in mind that they may worsen other side effects, such as cognition, constipation, and orthostatic hypotension (Praharaj et al., 2006; Spivak et al., 1997; Richardson et al., 2001; Webber et al., 2004). To avoid such side effects, atropine drops sublingually before sleep or as required during the day may alleviate the problem (Schneider et al., 2014; Mustafa et al., 2013). Amisulpride (Kreinin et al., 2006), sulpiride (Kreinin et al., 2005), and moclobemide (Kreinin et al., 2011) have also been suggested. In the most severe cases, injection of botulinum toxin into the parotid gland can reduce salivation, but this is limited in clinical settings by its invasive nature (Kahl et al., 2004).

Our focus is to ensure that hypersalivation only occurs during the night, as daytime hypersalivation is very stigmatizing for the patient. This can usually be done by giving the largest dose of clozapine at nighttime. Patients often have to accept nighttime hypersalivation as it is very difficult to address completely as plasma levels of clozapine peak after the nighttime dose, the supine position promotes hypersalivation, and the swallowing reflex is diminished during sleep. Because of the less systemic absorption, we recommend sublingual atropine drops before bedtime and during the day if necessary. In addition, even in cases where one anticholinergic medication has failed, it is our experience that others may succeed, so it is worth trying others. All interventions should be evaluated carefully because anticholinergics contribute significantly to the burden of side effects. A clozapine-sparing antipsychotic is often effective, as this may facilitate a dose reduction of clozapine.

Common (1-10%) adverse effects

Seizure risk

Clozapine increases the risk of seizures more than other antipsychotic drugs and alteration of electroencephalographic activity is common (Devinsky et al., 1991; Freudenreich et al., 1997). These effects are dose-dependent, and the risk of seizures in patients receiving more than 600 mg/day is 4.4% compared to 1.0% for patients receiving less than 300 mg/day, with a cumulative risk as high as 10% during 3.8 years of treatment; this emphasizes the importance of finding the lowest effective dose of clozapine (Devinsky et al., 1991).

Clozapine can cause different types of seizures, including tonic–clonic, myoclonic, simple, or complex partial seizures. It is important to exclude other reasons for seizure-like behaviour, including tardive dyskinesia or dissociative seizures, before considering a diagnosis of clozapine-induced seizure.

Before initiation of clozapine, it may be important to optimize other causes for decreased seizure threshold, including drugs causing seizures, alcohol or benzodiazepine withdrawal, organic brain disorders, electrolyte abnormalities, sleep deprivation, etc.

If the patient experiences a clozapine-induced seizure, clozapine should be discontinued for 24 hours and re-started at a lower dose (often a reduction of 50%) (Nielsen et al., 2013). Consider initiating a prophylactic antiepileptic such as sodium valproate or an alternative for women of childbearing potential (Williams and Park, 2015) (Table 7.2). Obtaining plasma levels of clozapine should be considered, as this can be used to exclude toxic levels of clozapine. Many clozapine-induced seizures occur as a consequence of a rapid increase in plasma levels owing to causes such as infections, smoking cessation, or administering a CYP1A2 inhibitor (Williams and Park, 2015).

Although many antiepileptic drugs have been used (gabapentin, lamotrigine, topiramate, phenytoin, and carbamazepine), the most extensive literature recommends valproate as first-line treatment. By reducing the dose of clozapine, slower dose titration, or addition of an antiepileptic drug, 78.3% of patients will not experience additional seizures (Williams and Park, 2015; Devinsky and Pacia, 1994) and seizures should therefore not lead to discontinuation of clozapine.

When we have patients experiencing seizures, we order clozapine plasma levels at first, discontinue clozapine for 24 hours, and re-start with a 50% lower dose and slowly up-titrate the dose guided by the clinical state and plasma levels. This is often enough, and most patients in our experience will not experience additional seizures. Often, our experience is that the seizures are related to an

Table 7.2 Management of common adverse effects of clozapine

Type	Management strategy	Discontinuation	Clinical comments
Seizures	Before clozapine initiation it is important to address other causes for decreased seizure threshold, e.g. alcohol or benzodiazepine withdrawal. *Treatment of clozapine-induced seizure:* Obtain plasma levels of clozapine and pause clozapine for 24 hours. Re-start at a lower dose (dose reduction of 50%) and consider prophylactic treatment with valproate. Other antiepileptic drugs (gabapentin, lamotrigine, topiramate, phenytoin, carbamazepine) can also be used and are advised for women of childbearing potential.	No reason for discontinuation.	Important to rule out causes of rapid increases in plasma levels of clozapine, such as infection, smoking cessation, or administration of CYP1A2 inhibitor.
Enuresis	*Non-pharmacological treatment:* Restriction of fluids before bedtime. Double voiding before bedtime. Avoiding caffeine and alcohol. *Pharmacological treatment:* Lowest effective clozapine dose. Lowest dose of clozapine at night (if other side effects do not prevent this). Drugs that can be used: desmopressin, anticholinergic drugs, ephedrine, tricyclic antidepressants, and add-on aripiprazole.	No reason for discontinuation.	Intranasal administration of desmopressin usually alleviates the problem. If patient continues drinking after desmopressin has been administered, a clozapine-sparing antipsychotic should be used instead.

ongoing infection or smoking cessation, leading to high plasma levels. Warning signs of seizure are usually myoclonic jerks, which should alert psychiatrists to focus on the risk of seizures.

If the mental status warrants high plasma levels or plasma levels that in this patient have been associated with a seizure, we recommend that prophylactic treatment with sodium valproate or, particularly in women of childbearing potential, another antiepileptic drug, is commenced. The use of clozapine-sparing antipsychotics should also be considered, especially when other dose-dependent side effects are present.

Enuresis

The exact mechanism of clozapine-induced enuresis remains largely unknown, but sedation, nighttime seizures, change in autonomic functions, secondary polyuria due to diabetes mellitus, or psychogenic polyuria may all contribute. Actively asking the patient about enuresis is important, as patients are often too embarrassed to report this adverse effect.

Non-pharmacological treatment includes restriction of fluids before bedtime, double voiding before bedtime, and avoiding caffeine and alcohol. Regarding pharmacological treatment, it is important to keep the dose of clozapine to the lowest effective dose and rearrange the dose by reducing the dose given at nighttime if other side effects such as sedation do not prevent this (Sagy et al., 2014). In addition, drugs such as desmopressin, tricyclic antidepressants, anticholinergic drugs, and ephedrine can be used, but no firm recommendation exists and many of these drugs may increase the risk of other serious adverse effects (Fuller et al., 1996; Steingard, 1994; Poyurovsky et al., 1996; Praharaj and Arora, 2007).

Our recommendation is to make sure that patients do not take fluids, caffeine, or alcohol after dinner. Normally this is enough to prevent nocturnal enuresis. If this is not the case, we prescribe intranasal desmopressin for the night. It is important to ensure that patients do not continue to drink after administration of desmopressin as this may be dangerous. In our experience, giving some of the clozapine dose during the day will in many cases lead to sedation, and we rarely succeed with this. The use of a non-sedating clozapine-sparing antipsychotic drug may also alleviate nocturnal enuresis.

Common cardiac adverse effects

Tachycardia and other cardiac adverse effects

Sinus tachycardia is a normal response to clozapine initiation and diminishes after 4–6 weeks of treatment. However, as clozapine has been linked to serious adverse effects such as myocarditis and neuroleptic malignant syndrome, which may have non-specific symptoms such as fever and tachycardia, it is important to exclude these conditions (Rohde et al., 2018). Normally, sinus tachycardia is not associated with any symptoms, and treatment should only be implemented if the tachycardia becomes symptomatic or severe. Treatment consists of beta-adrenergic antagonists (Stryjer et al., 2009). It is important to emphasize that sinus tachycardia is generally a benign phenomenon, which should not lead to discontinuation of clozapine (Table 7.3).

Non-specific ECG changes are a common finding during treatment with clozapine. This may include ST-segment changes, T-wave inversion, and T-wave

Table 7.3 Management of cardiac adverse effects of clozapine

Type	Management strategy	Discontinuation	Clinical comments
Sinus tachycardia	Normal response during the first 4–6 weeks of clozapine treatment. If it is symptomatic or severe, initiation of a cardioselective beta-adrenergic antagonist should be considered.	No reason for discontinuation. However, it is important to exclude other rare reasons, such as myocarditis and neuroleptic malignant syndrome.	Even if the patient is not presenting with palpitations, many patients will appreciate treatment with a beta-adrenergic antagonist.
Electrocardiogram abnormalities	Including ST-segment changes, T-wave inversion, and T-wave flattening.	No reason for discontinuation of clozapine if cardiac disease is excluded.	
QT-prolongation	Rare complication. Use the Fridericia formula if heart rate exceeds 80 bpm, as the Bazett formula only is valid for heart rates below 80 bpm (Nielsen et al., 2011). Manual electrocardiogram reading may be warranted	QTc >500 ms,	History of syncopes may warrant intervention even if QTc <500 ms,
Orthostatic hypotension	*Treatment:* Slow up-titration, increased fluids, and sufficient salt intake may diminish this complication. In severe cases, compression socks or low-dose fludrocortisone may help.	No reason for discontinuation,	

flattening (Kang et al., 2000). The ECG changes often only have minor clinical significance and discontinuation is not warranted if cardiac diseases are excluded. QT-prolongation should be mentioned as it is a commonly known adverse effect of many antipsychotic drugs. However, it is a rare adverse effect of clozapine and it may very well have been overestimated in early studies.

This is because normal QTc estimation is calculated by using Bazett's formula, which is only reliable at heart rates below 80 bpm. As clozapine is likely to induce tachycardia, as mentioned before, Bazett's formula overestimates the QTc interval, and the Fridericia formula offers a more appropriate QT correction in patients receiving clozapine. To avoid unnecessary discontinuation of clozapine owing to false QTc prolongation, it is therefore important to use the Fridericia formula if the heart rate exceeds 80 bpm (Nielsen et al., 2011). In addition, because of non-specific T-wave morphology it is important to read the ECG manually (Kang et al., 2000).

As a last common cardiac adverse effect of clozapine initiation, orthostatic hypotension should be mentioned. This is due to clozapine's noradrenergic alpha-1-receptor antagonistic effect, and it can be managed by using slow up-titration in combination with increased fluids and salt intake, supplemented in some cases with low-dose fludrocortisone (Nielsen et al., 2013; Low and Singer, 2008).

REFERENCES

Afshar H, Roohafza H, Mousavi G, et al. (2009). Topiramate add-on treatment in schizophrenia, a randomised, double-blind, placebo-controlled clinical trial. *J Psychopharmacol*, 23(2),157–62.

Bishara D, Taylor D. (2014). Adverse effects of clozapine in older patients: epidemiology, prevention and management. *Drugs Aging*, 31(1), 11–20.

Carrizo E, Fernandez V, Connell L, et al. (2009). Extended release metformin for metabolic control assistance during prolonged clozapine administration: a 14 week, double-blind, parallel group, placebo-controlled study. *Schizophr Res*, 113(1), 19–26.

Chen CH, Huang MC, Kao CF, et al. (2013). Effects of adjunctive metformin on metabolic traits in nondiabetic clozapine-treated patients with schizophrenia and the effect of metformin discontinuation on body weight: a 24-week, randomized, double-blind, placebo-controlled study. *J Clin Psychiatry*, 74(5), e424–30.

Costilla VC, Foxx-Orenstein AE. (2014). Constipation, understanding mechanisms and management. *Clin Geriatr Med*, 30(1), 107–15.

De Hert M, Detraux J, van Winkel R, Yu W, Correll CU. (2011). Metabolic and cardiovascular adverse effects associated with antipsychotic drugs. *Nature Reviews Endocrinol*, 8(2), 114–26.

de Leon J, Diaz FJ, Josiassen RC, Cooper TB, Simpson GM. (2007). Weight gain during a double-blind multidosage clozapine study. *J Clin Psychopharmacol*, 27(1), 22–7.

Devinsky O, Pacia SV. (1994). Seizures during clozapine therapy. *J Clin Psychiatry*, 55 (Suppl. B), 153–6.

Devinsky O, Honigfeld G, Patin J. (1991). Clozapine-related seizures. *Neurology*, 41(3), 369–71.

Edwards IR, Aronson JK. (2000). Adverse drug reactions, definitions, diagnosis, and management. *Lancet*, 356(9237), 1255–9.

Every-Palmer S, Newton-Howes G, Clarke MJ. (2017). Pharmacological treatment for antipsychotic-related constipation. *Schizophr Bull*, 2017, 43(3), 490–2.

Freudenreich O, Weiner RD, McEvoy JP. (1997). Clozapine-induced electroencephalogram changes as a function of clozapine serum levels. *Biol Psychiatry,* 42(2), 132–7.

Fuller MA, Borovicka MC, Jaskiw GE, Simon MR, Kwon K, Konicki PE. (1996). Clozapine-induced urinary incontinence, incidence and treatment with ephedrine. *J Clin Psychiatry,* 57(11), 514–18.

Hahn MK, Remington G, Bois D, Cohn T. (2010). Topiramate augmentation in clozapine-treated patients with schizophrenia: clinical and metabolic effects. *J Clin Psychopharmacol,* 30(6), 706–10.

Henderson DC, Kunkel L, Nguyen DD, et al. (2006). An exploratory open-label trial of aripiprazole as an adjuvant to clozapine therapy in chronic schizophrenia. *Acta Psychiatrica Scand,* 113(2), 142–7.

Kahl KG, Hagenah J, Zapf S, Trillenberg P, Klein C, Lencer R. (2004). Botulinum toxin as an effective treatment of clozapine-induced hypersalivation. *Psychopharmacology,* 173(1–2), 229–30.

Kane J, Honigfeld G, Singer J, Meltzer H. (1988). Clozapine for the treatment-resistant schizophrenic. A double-blind comparison with chlorpromazine. *Arch Gen Psychiatry,* 45(9), 789–96.

Kang UG, Kwon JS, Ahn YM, et al. (2000). Electrocardiographic abnormalities in patients treated with clozapine. *J Clin Psychiatry* 61(6), 441–6.

Kreinin A, Epshtein S, Sheinkman A, Tell E. (2005). Sulpiride addition for the treatment of clozapine-induced hypersalivation: preliminary study. *Israel J Psychiatry Rel Sci,* 42(1), 61–3.

Kreinin A, Novitski D, Weizman A. (2006). Amisulpride treatment of clozapine-induced hypersalivation in schizophrenia patients: a randomized, double-blind, placebo-controlled cross-over study. *Int Clin Psychopharmacol,* 21(2), 99–103.

Kreinin A, Miodownik C, Sokolik S, et al. (2011). Amisulpride versus moclobemide in treatment of clozapine-induced hypersalivation. *World J Biol Psychiatry,* 12(8), 620–6.

Larsen JR, Vedtofte L, Jakobsen MSL, et al. (2017). Effect of liraglutide treatment on prediabetes and overweight or obesity in clozapine- or olanzapine-treated patients with schizophrenia spectrum disorder: a randomized clinical trial. *JAMA Psychiatry,* 74(7), 719–28.

Low PA, Singer W. (2008). Management of neurogenic orthostatic hypotension: an update. *Lancet Neurol,* 7(5), 451–8.

Lu ML, Lane HY, Lin SK, Chen KP, Chang WH. (2004). Adjunctive fluvoxamine inhibits clozapine-related weight gain and metabolic disturbances. *J Clin Psychiatry,* 65(6), 766–71.

McEvoy JP, Lieberman JA, Stroup TS, et al. (2006). Effectiveness of clozapine versus olanzapine, quetiapine, and risperidone in patients with chronic schizophrenia who did not respond to prior atypical antipsychotic treatment. *Am J Psychiatry,* 163(4), 600–10.

Miller DD. (2000). Review and management of clozapine side effects. *J Clin Psychiatry,* 61 (Suppl. 8), 14–17, discussion 18–19.

Mustafa FA, Khan A, Burke J, Cox M, Sherif S. (2013). Sublingual atropine for the treatment of severe and hyoscine-resistant clozapine-induced sialorrhea. *African J Psychiatry,* 16(4), 242.

CHAPTER 7

Nielsen J, Graff C, Kanters JK, Toft E, Taylor D, Meyer JM. (2011). Assessing QT interval prolongation and its associated risks with antipsychotics. *CNS Drugs*, 25(6), 473–90.

Nielsen J, Nielsen RE, Correll CU. (2012). Predictors of clozapine response in patients with treatment-refractory schizophrenia: results from a Danish Register Study. *J Clin Psychopharmacol*, 32(5), 678–83.

Nielsen J, Correll CU, Manu P, Kane JM. (2013). Termination of clozapine treatment due to medical reasons: when is it warranted and how can it be avoided? *J Clin Psychiatry*, 74(6), 603–13, quiz 613.

Palmer SE, McLean RM, Ellis PM, Harrison-Woolrych M. (2008). Life-threatening clozapine-induced gastrointestinal hypomotility: an analysis of 102 cases. *J Clin Psychiatry*, 69(5), 759–68.

Perdigues SR, Quecuti RS, Mane A, Mann L, Mundell C, Fernandez-Egea E. (2016). An observational study of clozapine induced sedation and its pharmacological management. *European Neuropsychopharmacol* 26(1), 156–61.

Poyurovsky M, Modai I, Weizman A. (1996). Trihexyphenidyl as a possible therapeutic option in clozapine-induced nocturnal enuresis. *Int Clin Psychopharmacol*, 11(1), 61–3.

Praharaj SK, Arora M. (2007). Amitriptyline for clozapine-induced nocturnal enuresis and sialorrhoea. *Br J Clin Pharmacol*, 63(1), 128–9.

Praharaj SK, Arora M, Gandotra S. (2006). Clozapine-induced sialorrhea, pathophysiology and management strategies. *Psychopharmacology*, 185(3), 265–73.

Richardson C, Kelly DL, Conley RR. (2001). Biperiden for excessive sweating from clozapine. *Am J Psychiatry*, 158(8), 1329–30.

Rohde C, Polcwiartek C, Asztalos M, Nielsen J. (2018). Effectiveness of prescription-based CNS stimulants on hospitalization in patients with schizophrenia: a nation-wide register study. *Schizophr Bull*, 44(1), 93–100.

Rohde C, Polcwiartek C, Kragholm K, Ebdrup BH, Siskind D, Nielsen J. (2018). Adverse cardiac events in out-patients initiating clozapine treatment: a nationwide register-based study. *Acta Psychiatrica Scandinavica*, 137(1), 47–53.

Sagy R, Weizman A, Katz N. (2014). Pharmacological and behavioral management of some often-overlooked clozapine-induced side effects. *Int Clin Psychopharmacol*, 29(6), 313–17.

Schneider C, Corrigall R, Hayes D, Kyriakopoulos M, Frangou S. (2014). Systematic review of the efficacy and tolerability of clozapine in the treatment of youth with early onset schizophrenia. *Eur Psychiatry*, 29(1), 1–10.

Shirazi A, Stubbs B, Gomez L, et al. (2016). Prevalence and predictors of clozapine-associated constipation: a systematic review and meta-analysis. *Int J Mol Sci*, 17(6), 863.

Spivak B, Adlersberg S, Rosen L, Gonen N, Mester R, Weizman A. (1997). Trihexyphenidyl treatment of clozapine-induced hypersalivation. *Int Clin Psychopharmacol*, 12(4), 213–15.

Steingard S. (1994). Use of desmopressin to treat clozapine-induced nocturnal enuresis. *J Clin Psychiatry*, 55(7), 315–16.

Stryjer R, Timinsky I, Reznik I, Weizman A, Spivak B. (2009). Beta-adrenergic antagonists for the treatment of clozapine-induced sinus tachycardia: a retrospective study. *Clin Neuropharmacol*, 32(5), 290–2.

Webber MA, Szwast SJ, Steadman TM, et al. (2004). Guanfacine treatment of clozapine-induced sialorrhea. *J Clin Psychopharmacol,* 24(6), 675–6.

Whitney Z, Procyshyn RM, Fredrikson DH, Barr AM. (2015). Treatment of clozapine-associated weight gain: a systematic review. *Eur J Clin Pharmacol,* 71(4), 389–401.

Williams AM, Park SH. (2015). Seizure associated with clozapine: incidence, etiology, and management. *CNS Drugs,* 29(2), 101–11.

Wu MK, Wang CK, Bai YM, Huang CY, Lee SD. (2007). Outcomes of obese, clozapine-treated inpatients with schizophrenia placed on a six-month diet and physical activity program. *Psychiatric Services,* 58(4), 544–50.

Young CR, Bowers MB, Jr., Mazure CM. (1998). Management of the adverse effects of clozapine. *Schizophr Bull,* 1998, 24(3), 381–90.

CHAPTER 8

Pharmacological management of treatment-resistant schizophrenia: advanced use of clozapine

Siobhan Gee and David Taylor

> **KEY POINTS**
>
> - Clozapine is licensed in many countries for use in treatment-resistant schizophrenia, treatment-intolerant schizophrenia, or psychosis associated with Parkinson's disease.
> - As with many drugs, it is also used outside of these licensing parameters for other conditions or clinical situations, such as for aggression, mood disorders, or in children. This is referred to as 'off-label' prescribing.
> - These off-label indications have varying degrees of theoretical support, peer-reviewed evidence, and practical experience associated with them.
> - Clozapine can be effectively used in children and older adults with adaptation.
> - Clozapine can also be effective for aggression and mood disorders.
> - The use of supramaximal doses of clozapine to achieve therapeutic plasma concentrations is also off-label, although adding interacting medication to reach the same result is not; these contrasting approaches are also debated.
> - Clozapine can be re-started after serious events such as neutropenia and myocarditis but with additional precautions.

Children and adolescents

Of these 'off-label' uses, prescribing of clozapine to children (under 16 years old) is perhaps the most controversial. The use of a potentially dangerous medication in young people is inevitably worrying, but so is the potential long-term impact of undertreating early-onset schizophrenia. Very early-onset schizophrenia (diagnosed before age 13) and adolescent-onset schizophrenia may be particularly associated with more severe symptoms, poorer clinical and social outcomes, and a high rate of antipsychotic resistance (Schneider et al., 2015). Clozapine is effective in children (Schneider et al., 2014) and is recommended by the UK National Institute for Health and Care Excellence (NICE) for use where the illness has not responded to two different antipsychotic treatments, in the same way as for adult patients.

Published experience of using clozapine in children and adolescents in trial settings originates largely from the USA, where dosing that is analogous to adult dosing is used (starting at 12.5 mg/day, increasing every 2–3 days in 12.5–25-mg increments according to response). Most patients respond to a target dose of 350–550 mg/day (Gogtay and Rapoport, 2008). Measuring plasma concentrations may be helpful, in the same way as for adults, although small studies have suggested that adolescents may generate proportionately more norclozapine (Piscitelli et al., 1994), and so the ratio of clozapine to norclozapine may be a more useful predictor of response. Plasma concentrations of clozapine are proportionately associated with side effects in children (Wohkittel et al., 2016) and are influenced by similar variables to those observed in adults (Couchman et al., 2013), and so are likely to be valuable in establishing tolerability as well as efficacy.

Children may be more susceptible to the adverse effects of clozapine than adults (Gogtay and Rapoport, 2008). The most common side effects reported are sedation and hypersalivation, with enuresis, constipation, and weight gain also frequently reported (Schneider et al., 2014). Prescribers should be mindful of the long-term impact of weight gain and dyslipidaemia and monitor carefully, intervening to prevent weight gain as early as possible.

Older people

At the other end of the spectrum, there is no obvious reason to suspect that clozapine would be less effective than other medications in the treatment of psychosis in elderly patients (and this is a licensed indication). Indeed, it may be a more appropriate antipsychotic choice than any other, given the increased risk of extrapyramidal side effects with advancing age. As with all drug treatments, careful consideration should be made of likely additional comorbidities, changes in drug handling parameters, and concurrent medications. Older patients are generally more susceptible to adverse effects of medication; of particular note is the hypotensive effect of clozapine, which may pose a risk to the frail elderly, especially if other antihypertensive treatments are co-prescribed. Constipation and urinary retention may also be problematic. Starting at low doses (6.25–12.5 mg/day) and titrating more gradually (over weeks or months) is a sensible approach, and prescribers should note that the maintenance dose required is likely to be lower than that in younger adults (average doses are 50–100 mg/day, although higher doses may be required in those who have become 'old' whilst on clozapine) (Bishara and Taylor, 2014). Doses in this lower range have been shown to achieve plasma concentrations in the therapeutic range (0.35–0.5 mg/L), probably owing to decreased clearance of clozapine and norclozapine in older age (Bowskill et al., 2012). Even lower doses (6.25–50 mg/day) can be used to treat psychosis in Parkinson's disease. Clozapine is an obvious antipsychotic choice in this circumstance because of its low propensity to cause extrapyramidal side effects, and many open label studies as well as some double-blind randomized controlled trials have confirmed efficacy and tolerability (Frieling et al., 2007; Parkinson Study Group, 1999; Wilby et al., 2017). The fact that clozapine is so effective at such low doses suggests perhaps a different mode of action than in schizophrenia.

Aggression

Clozapine is known to have antiaggressive effects in both adults and adolescents suffering psychosis (Frogley et al., 2012). Data regarding its ability to reduce violent behaviour in other diagnostic groups are less clear. Antiaggressive effects appear to be greater than simply the antipsychotic or sedative properties of the drug; the mechanism of action may be related to anxiolytic effects mediated by activity at 5-HT2A or 5-HT1A receptors. This is suggested in part because the magnitude of reduction in violence appears to be greater than concomitant reduction in psychotic symptoms, and is observed to be temporally unrelated. Additionally, animal studies have shown that the antiaggressive effect is independent of sedation, but not of locomotor activity, again pointing to an antianxiety effect. The serotonergic system has long been thought to be of particular relevance in the pathophysiology of violent behaviour, and of course clozapine is somewhat unusual amongst antipsychotics in binding to 5-HT receptors as well as dopaminergic receptors.

The evidence base for the use of clozapine off-label to reduce aggression in non-psychotic patients is limited to small open-label studies and case reports. Some suggest superiority of clozapine compared to other antipsychotics in reduction of aggression in people with autism spectrum disorders (Beherec et al., 2011; Lambrey et al., 2010). Further reports describe antiaggressive effects in other conditions, including borderline personality disorder, impulse control disorder, post-traumatic stress disorder, and learning disability (Kraus and Sheitman, 2005; Frogley et al., 2012).

Beyond a reduction in aggressive incidents (both to others and themselves), clozapine may also benefit those with borderline personality disorder in terms of symptom severity, the need for enhanced observations, and the use of additional medication (Frogley et al., 2013). This may also be achievable at lower doses and plasma levels than usually required in psychosis spectrum disorders (25–100 mg/day) (Benedetti et al., 1998). It is possible that this effect is also mediated via anxiolytic effects, considered to be of particular importance in borderline personality disorder.

Mood disorders

The 'mood-stabilizing' and anxiolytic effect of clozapine has also been explored in trials examining use in patients with bipolar affective disorder. In naturalistic studies, patients with bipolar disorders required lower doses than those with schizophrenia for symptom reduction (around 150 mg/day) and were more likely than those with schizophrenia to derive significant improvement not only in symptoms but also in occupational domains. They were additionally less likely to discontinue treatment and had shorter times to remission (Ciapparelli et al., 2003). It may be relevant to consider the predominant polarity of symptoms requiring treatment; patients with bipolar mania or schizomanic disorders appear to gain more benefit from treatment with clozapine than their counterparts with schizophrenia or schizoaffective depressive disorders (McElroy et al., 1991). It may be that this is due to the manic part of the illness responding particularly well to clozapine, even at low doses (Aksoy Poyraz et al., 2015; Calabrese et al., 1996; Fehr et al., 2005; Suppes et al., 1999).

There is growing support for the use of clozapine in bipolar disorder, with some UK guidelines recommending use off-label (Box 8.1) in refractory or rapid cycling illness (Goodwin and Consensus Group for the British Association for Psychopharmacology, 2009), although the evidence base is still limited to two randomized controlled trials and several retrospective studies, open-label trials, and case reports. Clozapine can be added to lithium or anticonvulsant treatment or used as monotherapy, and a comprehensive systematic review (which included Chinese data, where clozapine is widely used as a first-line treatment in bipolar disorder) found it to be safe and effective (Li et al., 2015). The additional benefits of clozapine in reduction in suicide risk (Meltzer et al., 2003) should not be forgotten when considering treatment choice in a condition with a high lifetime risk of completed suicide.

Clozapine rapid metabolizers

In some ways, it is unfortunate that the licence for the dose of clozapine describes a range of milligrams to be given per day, rather than a plasma level to be attained. It is widely accepted that a plasma level of 0.35–0.5 mg/L is required for minimal clinical efficacy, but for patients who are rapid metabolizers of clozapine, are taking interacting medications, or are heavy smokers, this therapeutic range

---

Box 8.1 Prescribing off-label

'Off-label' prescribing refers to the prescribing of a licensed medication for an unlicensed indication

Familiarize yourself with the available evidence for the proposed unlicensed indication, including potential adverse effects. Discuss with expert colleagues where possible

Consider carefully the risks and benefits of such a treatment

Discuss the proposed treatment plan with the patient and carer(s) where possible, and document this discussion in the clinical notes

Monitor closely for effectiveness and adverse effects

Stop the treatment if it proves ineffective

Consider publishing the case

---

may be difficult to achieve whilst remaining within the licensed dose boundaries. If therapeutic plasma concentrations cannot be reached at the maximum licensed dose per day (900 mg) then three options are available to clinicians:

1. Abandon efforts to achieve therapeutic plasma concentrations of clozapine and instead either switch to a non-clozapine antipsychotic regimen, or augment the subtherapeutic clozapine with another drug (commonly a second antipsychotic).
2. Increase the dose beyond the licensing boundaries (>900 mg/day) to achieve therapeutic plasma levels.
3. Use an interacting drug to inhibit the metabolism of clozapine and boost the plasma levels to within the therapeutic range.

None of these approaches is without risk. Adding a second antipsychotic to clozapine inevitably compounds side effects and is without a clear evidence base to support efficacy (Taylor et al., 2012). Increasing the dose beyond the licensed maximum is possible but, if metabolism is rapid, this may simply increase the levels of metabolites and attendant side effects, with little appreciable increase in clozapine levels. Furthermore, dose increases, even within the licensed range, may be unacceptable to patients because of the increased tablet burden. Although this strategy is unlicensed, the increase in plasma levels achieved may be considered more predictable than the alternative approach of adding an interacting drug.

Fluvoxamine, a selective serotonin reuptake inhibitor and potent CYP1A2 inhibitor, has been used to alter the metabolic processing of clozapine, increasing clozapine plasma concentrations and lowering norclozapine concentrations (Polcwiartek and Nielsen, 2016). This latter effect is of particular interest for patients who are struggling to tolerate therapeutic plasma concentrations of clozapine, as the metabolites are known to act on different receptor systems to the parent drug and may be responsible for different tolerability problems. It has been additionally suggested that the ratio of clozapine to norclozapine may be of relevance for efficacy (although this has not yet been characterized). Cimetidine is a histamine receptor antagonist and a moderately potent multienzyme inhibitor. It is also an inhibitor of CYP1A2, but to a lesser extent than fluvoxamine. Case reports (Watras and Taylor, 2013) describe its addition to clozapine, resulting in a 1.9-fold increase in clozapine plasma levels (compared with a 5–12-fold increase associated with fluvoxamine).

Caution with this approach is warranted. The magnitude of the effects on clozapine and norclozapine plasma concentrations appears highly variable and unpredictable. Clinicians should be aware that, although the effect of adjunctive fluvoxamine on clozapine plasma levels is dose-dependent, fluvoxamine displays non-linear pharmacokinetics at doses above 50 mg per day, potentially increasing clozapine levels in an unpredictable manner. The consequences of a sudden rise in clozapine plasma levels may be profound hypotension, tachycardia, sedation, and

> **Box 8.2** Adding an augmenting agent to clozapine to increase plasma levels
>
> • Titrate the augmenting agent slowly, from a low starting dose (25 mg fluvoxamine)
> • Measure clozapine and norclozapine plasma levels after each dose increase of the augmenting agent, allowing at least 10 days of stable dosing before taking a clozapine plasma level
> • Only increase doses after obtaining repeat clozapine and norclozapine plasma levels
> • Monitor carefully for dose-dependent adverse effects of clozapine

seizures. There may be additional benefits to be gained from augmenting in this way, beyond purely increased plasma levels of clozapine (fluvoxamine may help to treat negative or depressive symptoms, and gastro-oesophageal reflux disease is disproportionately common in patients taking clozapine) (Box 8.2).

Re-starting clozapine after neutropenia or other serious adverse events

Whilst clozapine is associated with a wide range of adverse effects, most are either treatable or at least modifiable to an extent sufficient to allow safe and tolerable continued treatment. Some side effects, however, warrant immediate cessation of therapy; these include profound neutropenia, agranulocytosis, and myocarditis. These conditions, or other similarly serious scenarios, may also arise during treatment with non-clozapine antipsychotics. Clozapine's unique place in the treatment of schizophrenia where all other drugs have failed means that clinicians may find themselves considering re-starting clozapine for such patients where, in the case of other drugs, the offending agent would likely be discarded from future treatment options.

Neutropenia may be secondary to factors other than clozapine treatment and, before considering rechallenge, these must be carefully considered. Benign ethnic neutropenia (BEN) affects up to 25% of those of African and Middle Eastern ancestry (Meyer et al., 2015). For these patients, the neutropenia may not be clozapine-related and so diagnosis of BEN allows the use of modified monitoring parameters for white blood cells, hopefully leading to uninterrupted continued treatment. If reduction of the acceptable threshold for white blood cells is insufficient to ensure that neutrophils remain above agreed cut-off points, then treatment with lithium or granulocyte-colony stimulating factors may be considered. It is important to note that both of these options do not protect the patient from a drug-induced neutropenia—they only raise baseline levels of measurable neutrophils, allowing continued clozapine treatment where patients would otherwise be required to discontinue clozapine owing to low congenital white cell counts. As such, they should be used with caution, and only if prescribers can be certain that the previous neutropenia was not clozapine-induced. Coadministration of lithium during clozapine rechallenge in patients with previous non-clozapine-induced neutropenia increases the likelihood of a successful outcome from around 40% to almost 95% (Manu et al., 2012), making this a worthwhile strategy. Other causes of non-clozapine-induced neutropenia include coadministration of medicines such as sodium valproate (Malik et al., 2018); these treatments should be discontinued before attempting clozapine rechallenge. In all cases, more frequent blood testing (twice-weekly) is advisable, ideally for the first 3 months of treatment, to identify any recurrence of neutropenia quickly (which may occur more rapidly than experienced previously).

For patients who have experienced clozapine-induced agranulocytosis, the outcome following rechallenge is much less likely to be positive (as many as 80% of patients may have a recurrence of agranulocytosis) (Manu et al., 2012). Treatments such as lithium and granulocyte-colony stimulating factors cannot protect from such an event, and these patients should probably not be rechallenged with clozapine.

Myocarditis, a hypersensitivity reaction to clozapine that results in inflammation of the myocardium, is most likely to occur in the first 8 weeks of starting clozapine (but may arise at any time), and is potentially fatal. Should it occur, immediate treatment cessation is essential. Confirmation of the diagnosis is often challenging—many of the symptoms of myocarditis are seen in patients who do not have the condition and, conversely, the absence of symptoms does not necessarily rule out myocarditis. Patients with suspected myocarditis should be referred to a cardiologist for an echocardiogram and (ideally) endomyocardial biopsy. A handful of case reports describes successful rechallenges (Chow et al., 2014; Manu et al., 2012) but data are insufficient to support this strategy confidently. The use of beta-blockers and angiotensin-converting enzyme inhibitors may help (Floreani and Bastiampillai, 2008). Weekly monitoring of troponin, C-reactive protein, and echocardiography is essential as recurrence is possible.

Conclusions

Clozapine is a potentially effective drug not only for patients with treatment-resistant schizophrenia or psychosis in Parkinson's disease, but for those suffering other mental health conditions, including mood disorders and situations not covered in its licence, such as children and patients who have experienced neutropenia. As with all drugs and indications, but especially those that may be unusual or for which the drug in question is not usually indicated, the evidence base is constantly evolving and expanding, and clinicians must therefore ensure that they are familiar with the available information and how it applies to their patient. It is always advisable to consult as many sources as possible, including peer-reviewed journal articles and expert consensus guidelines and textbooks, and experienced colleagues, both within the psychiatric field (including expert pharmacists) and without (for example, haematologists and cardiologists).

REFERENCES

Aksoy Poyraz, C., Turan, Ş., Demirel, Ö., Usta Sağlam, N., Yıldız, N., Duran, A. (2015). Effectiveness of ultra- rapid dose titration of clozapine for treatment- resistant bipolar mania: case series. *Ther Adv Psychopharmacol*, 5(4), 237–42.

Beherec, L., Lambrey, S., Quilici, G., Rosier, A., Falissard, B., Guillin, O. (2011). Retrospective review of clozapine in the treatment of patients with autism spectrum disorder and severe disruptive behaviors. *J Clin Psychopharmacol*, 31(3), 341–4.

Benedetti, F., Sforzini, L., Colombo, C., Maffei, C., Smeraldi, E. (1998). Low-dose clozapine in acute and continuation treatment of severe borderline personality disorder. *J Clin Psychiatry*, 59(3), 103–7.

Bishara, D., Taylor, D. (2014). Adverse effects of clozapine in older patients: epidemiology, prevention and management. *Drugs Aging*, 31(1), 11–20.

Bowskill, S., Couchman, L., MacCabe, J. H., Flanagan, R. J. (2012). Plasma clozapine and norclozapine in relation to prescribed dose and other factors in patients aged 65 years and over: data from a therapeutic drug monitoring service, 1996–2010. *Human Psychopharmacology: Clinical and Experimental*, 27(3), 277–83.

Calabrese, J., Kimmel, S., Woyshville, M., et al. (1996). Clozapine for treatment-refractory mania. *Am J Psychiatry*, 153(6), 759–64.

Chow, V., Feijo, I., Trieu, J., Starling, J., Kritharides, L. (2014). Successful rechallenge of clozapine therapy following previous clozapine-induced myocarditis confirmed on cardiac MRI. *J Child Adolesc Psychopharmacol*, 24(2), 99–101.

Ciapparelli, A., Dell'Osso, L., Di Poggio, A., et al. (2003). Clozapine in treatment-resistant patients with schizophrenia, schizoaffective disorder, or psychotic bipolar disorder: a naturalistic 48-month follow-up study. *J Clin Psychiatry*, 64(4), 451–8.

Couchman, L., Bowskill, S., Handley, S., Patel, M., Flanagan, R. (2013). Plasma clozapine and norclozapine in relation to prescribed dose and other factors in patients aged less than 18 years: data from a therapeutic drug monitoring service, 1994–2010. *Early Interv Psychiatry*, 7(2), 122–30.

Fehr, B. S., Ozcan, M. E., Suppes, T. (2005). Low doses of clozapine may stabilize treatment-resistant bipolar patients. *Eur Arch Psychiatry Clin Neurosci*, 255(1), 10–14.

Floreani, J., Bastiampillai, T. (2008). Successful re-challenge with clozapine following development of clozapine-induced cardiomyopathy. *Aust New Zealand J Psychiatry*, 42(8), 747–748. Retrieved from http://www.ncbi.nlm.nih.gov/pubmed/18642408

Frieling, H., Hillemacher, T., Ziegenbein, M., Neundorfer, B., Bleich, S. (2007). Treating dopamimetic psychosis in Parkinson's disease: structured review and meta-analysis. *Eur Neuropsychopharmacol*, 17(3), 165–171.

Frogley, C., Taylor, D., Dickens, G., Picchioni, M. (2012). A systematic review of the evidence of clozapine's anti-aggressive effects. *Int J Neuropsychopharmacol*, 15(9), 1351–71.

Frogley, C., Anagnostakis, K., Mitchell, S., et al. (2013). A case series of clozapine for borderline personality disorder. *Ann Clin Psychiatry*, 25(2), 125–34.

Gogtay, N., Rapoport, J. (2008). Clozapine use in children and adolescents. *Expert Opin Pharmacother*, 9(3), 459–65.

Goodwin, G., Consensus Group for the British Association for Psychopharmacology. (2009). Evidence-based guidelines for treating bipolar disorder: revised second edition—recommendations from the British Association for Psychopharmacology. *J Psychopharmacol*, 23(4), 346–88.

Kraus, J., Sheitman, B. (2005). Clozapine reduces violent behavior in heterogeneous diagnostic groups. *J Neuropsychiatry Clin Neurosci*, 17, 36–44.

Lambrey, S., Falissard, B., Martin-Barrero, M., et al. (2010). Effectiveness of clozapine for the treatment of aggression in an adolescent with autistic disorder. *J Child Adolesc Psychopharmacol*, 20(1), 79–80.

Li, X.-B., Tang, Y.-L., Wang, C.-Y., de Leon, J. (2015). Clozapine for treatment-resistant bipolar disorder: a systematic review. *Bipolar Disorders*, 17(3), 235–47.

Malik, S., Lally, J., Ajnakina, O., et al. (2018). Sodium valproate and clozapine induced neutropenia: a case control study using register data. *Schizophr Res*, 195, 267–73.

Manu, P., Sarpal, D., Muir, O., Kane, J. M., Correll, C. U. (2012). When can patients with potentially life-threatening adverse effects be rechallenged with clozapine? A systematic review of the published literature. *Schizophr Res*, 134(2–3), 180–6.

McElroy, S., Dessain, E., Pope, H., et al. (1991). Clozapine in the treatment of psychotic mood disorders, schizoaffective disorder, and schizophrenia. *J Clin Psychiatry*, 52(10), 411–14.

Meltzer, H., Alphs, L., Green, A., et al. and International Suicide Prevention Trial Study Group. (2003). Clozapine treatment for suicidality in schizophrenia: International Suicide Prevention Trial (InterSePT). *Arch Gen Psychiatry*, 60(1), 82–91.

Meyer, N., Gee, S., Whiskey, E., et al. (2015). Optimizing outcomes in clozapine rechallenge following neutropenia: a cohort analysis. *J Clin Psychiatry*, 76(11), e1410–16.

Parkinson Study Group. (1999). Low-dose clozapine for the treatment of drug-induced psychosis in Parkinson's disease. *New Engl J Med*, 340(10), 757–63. https://doi.org/10.1056/NEJM199903113401003

Piscitelli, S., Frazier, J., McKenna, K., et al. (1994). Plasma clozapine and haloperidol concentrations in adolescents with childhood-onset schizophrenia: association with response. *J Clin Psychiatry*, 55 (Suppl. B), 94–7.

Polcwiartek, C., Nielsen, J. (2016). The clinical potentials of adjunctive fluvoxamine to clozapine treatment: a systematic review. *Psychopharmacology*, 233(5), 741–50.

Schneider, C., Corrigall, R., Hayes, D., Kyriakopoulos, M., Frangou, S. (2014). Systematic review of the efficacy and tolerability of clozapine in the treatment of youth with early onset schizophrenia. *Eur Psychiatry*, 29(1), 1–10.

Schneider, C., Papachristou, E., Wimberley, T., et al. (2015). Clozapine use in childhood and adolescent schizophrenia: a nationwide population-based study. *Eur Neuropsychopharmacol*, 25(6), 857–63.

Suppes, T., Webb, A., Paul, B., Carmody, T., Kraemer, H., Rush, A. J. (1999). Clinical outcome in a randomized 1-year trial of clozapine versus treatment as usual for patients with treatment-resistant illness and a history of mania. *Am J Psychiatry*, 156(8), 1164–9.

Taylor, D., Smith, L., Gee, S., Nielsen, J. (2012). Augmentation of clozapine with a second antipsychotic—a meta-analysis. *Acta Psych Scand*, 125(1), 15–24.

Watras, M., Taylor, D. (2013). A therapeutic interaction between cimetidine and clozapine: case study and review of the literature. *Ther Adv Psychopharmacol*, 3(5), 294–7.

Wilby, K. J., Johnson, E. G., Johnson, H. E., Ensom, M. H. H. (2017). Evidence-based review of pharmacotherapy used for Parkinson's disease psychosis. *Ann Pharmacotherapy*, 51(8), 682–695.

Wohkittel, C., Gerlach, M., Taurines, R., et al. (2016). Relationship between clozapine dose, serum concentration, and clinical outcome in children and adolescents in clinical practice. *J Neural Transm*, 123(8), 1021–31.

CHAPTER 9

Pharmacological management of treatment-resistant schizophrenia: alternatives to clozapine

Thomas R. E. Barnes

KEY POINTS

- Other than clozapine, there are no pharmacological interventions with robust evidence of a positive benefit–risk balance for the treatment of resistant schizophrenia.

- For patients with a treatment-resistant illness, typically defined as failure to respond sufficiently to at least two adequate trials of standard antipsychotic medication, it would seem that there is usually little to be gained from a further switch of antipsychotic medication or the prescription of high-dose or combined antipsychotic medications.

- There is little evidence to support the augmentation of continuing antipsychotic medication with other medications, such as antidepressants, mood stabilizers, or benzodiazepines.

- In clinical practice, such augmentation strategies may be used to treat particular key symptoms or behaviours rather than to enhance the overall therapeutic efficacy of the medication regimen, although the evidence for such targeted benefit is largely lacking.

- In clinical practice, each initiation of high-dose or combined antipsychotic medication or an augmentation strategy should be treated as an individual trial and appropriately monitored and reviewed, with discontinuation in case of inefficacy or benefit that is outweighed by safety or tolerability concerns.

Introduction

Clozapine is the only antipsychotic for which there is robust and consistent evidence of efficacy in strictly defined, treatment-resistant schizophrenia (TRS); that is, illness that has failed to show a sufficient response to adequate trials of standard antipsychotic medication (Kane et al., 1988; Siskind et al., 2016). As the definition of TRS usually refers to persistent positive symptoms, it is for the treatment of such symptoms that clozapine appears to have superior efficacy. Despite some promising findings, whether clozapine has superior efficacy for persistent negative symptoms remains uncertain (Souza et al., 2013; Asenjo Lobos et al., 2010). There is also evidence suggesting that clozapine is clinically superior to other antipsychotic medication for treating persistent hostility and aggression in established schizophrenia (Frogley et al., 2012) and reducing the risk of suicide (Meltzer et al., 2003; Tiihonen et al., 2009a). However, when comparing clinical outcomes in patients prescribed clozapine in real-world practice with those continuing on other antipsychotic medications (Tiihonen et al., 2009a; Ringbäck Weitoft et al., 2014), it should be borne in mind that the former group is likely to be highly selected in terms of their lack of serious emergent side effects, their good cooperation with haematological monitoring and medication adherence (Ringbäck Weitoft et al., 2014) and a positive risk–benefit balance for clozapine in that, without evident therapeutic benefit that outweighs the potentially serious risks, it is unlikely that this medication would have been continued.

Alternatives to clozapine will be considered by clinicians for patients who have a diagnosis of TRS but have not yet been exposed to a trial of clozapine, perhaps because it is contraindicated or because, having explained the risks and benefits of the medication, the patient has declined it. Alternatives will also be considered where a trial of clozapine has failed, for whatever reason. An adequate trial of clozapine will not be feasible for all patients with a treatment-resistant illness. Some patients will be reluctant to comply with the mandatory haematological monitoring while, for others, the emergence of serious side effects will prevent the optimum dosage being achieved or will necessitate stopping the medication. Even when an adequate trial of clozapine is possible, for up to 40% of cases the response will be insufficient (Kontaxakis et al., 2005), although this may partly reflect that there has been too long a delay between the diagnosis of TRS and the initiation of clozapine (Yoshimura et al., 2017).

Currently there are no alternative pharmacological interventions with the same convincing level of evidence for efficacy for TRS as clozapine. Of the treatment strategies used clinically, switching antipsychotic medication, high-dose antipsychotic medication, and combined antipsychotic medication (antipsychotic polypharmacy) are probably the most common. Most of the alternative treatment strategies involve augmentation of continuing antipsychotic medication with a range of other medications, many of which are chosen because of claims that they can tackle particular symptoms or behaviours. TRS has a heterogeneous presentation and, rather than seek a treatment to achieve overall improvement, clinicians may target key symptoms that are distressing, disabling, or constitute a barrier to engagement with psychological and psychosocial interventions.

Switching to another antipsychotic medication

Changing the antipsychotic medication that is currently being administered is a common strategy when the response has been poor, but it is uncertain whether this is an effective strategy. If a trial of clozapine has proved ineffective or failed for some other reason, the question is which other antipsychotic should be given

(Dold and Leucht, 2014). Switching to another second-generation antipsychotic (SGA) medication, such as olanzapine or risperidone, has been recommended (Hasan et al., 2012), but meta-analyses of data from randomized trials reveal only modest differences in efficacy between the available non-clozapine antipsychotic medications (Leucht et al., 2013). However, much of this evidence is derived from samples of patients with a non-resistant illness and there must be doubts about the extent to which it is valid to extrapolate the findings to treatment-resistant illness. A network analysis of studies testing available antipsychotics in TRS concluded that the evidence was insufficient to determine which antipsychotic medication might be more efficacious (Samara et al., 2016).

Further, switching antipsychotic medication is not without its risks. These include destabilization of the illness and the induction of adverse effects, problems that may be attributable to stopping the current antipsychotic medication and/ or a response to the subsequent medication and/or differences between the pharmacological profiles of the two medications (Lambert, 2007). To minimize such potential complications, a gradual cross-tapering approach is usually recommended (Weiden, 2006; Lambert, 2007), although how the switch is managed in terms of immediate or gradual withdrawal of the current medication seems to have little clinical impact (Takeuchi et al., 2017).

For first-episode patients, early non-response to antipsychotic medication is a robust predictor of subsequent non-response (Stauffer et al., 2011; Lally et al., 2016). In a naturalistic study, Agid et al. (2011) followed a treatment algorithm in first-episode patients of two sequential trials of SGA medications (olanzapine followed by risperidone or vice versa), followed by clozapine. With the first antipsychotic trial, 75% of the sample met predefined response criteria, which reinforces previous findings of a high proportion of clinical responders with such medication in first-episode illness. However, when the patients in the subgroup with a poor response to the first antipsychotic medication were switched to the second antipsychotic, fewer than 20% responded. Of the patients whose illness failed to respond to both SGA trials and who subsequently agreed to a trial of clozapine, 75% showed a marked and significant improvement. While confirming the superiority of clozapine for TRS, the findings also show a limited value for switching to non-clozapine antipsychotic medications for the majority of patients with such an illness.

A similar conclusion may be drawn from the second phase of the Clinical Antipsychotic Trials of Intervention Effectiveness (CATIE) study (McEvoy et al., 2006), involving patients with established schizophrenia rather than in the early stages of the illness. A sample of the participants who had discontinued treatment with an SGA in the first phase of the CATIE study because of inefficacy was randomly assigned to treatment with either clozapine or another SGA that they had not previously received in the trial. The time to 'all-cause discontinuation' of the assigned treatment was significantly longer for clozapine than for quetiapine or risperidone, although not for olanzapine. This and other findings in the study led the investigators to conclude that, for schizophrenia with an inadequate response to SGA medication, switching to clozapine was more effective than switching to another SGA.

High-dose antipsychotic medication

The 'near-maximal effective dose' for an antipsychotic medication is the threshold dose necessary for all or almost all clinical response. The implication is that increasing the dose above this threshold would lead to a greater side effect burden without any additional clinical benefit. When Davis and Chen (2004) calculated this near-maximal effective dose for many of the available antipsychotic medications, they found that it was generally below what would be considered as a high dose and concluded that there was little or no evidence that doses higher than the near-maximal effective dose were more effective, generally or for TRS (Davis and Chen, 2004; Gardner et al., 2010).

Several studies have directly compared the efficacy of increasing antipsychotic dosage with maintaining the same dose in the treatment of people with schizophrenia that has shown a poor response to an initial antipsychotic drug trial. A meta-analysis of five such trials found no differences between the dose escalation and control groups in positive and negative symptom change scores, response rates, or drop-out rates (Dold et al., 2015). Similarly, another meta-analysis of such studies found not a single one in favour of the dose increase strategy (Helfer et al., 2015; Samara and Leucht, 2016). A Canadian Agency for Drugs and Technologies in Health report (2011) identified two relevant studies: high- versus standard-dose quetiapine for persistent symptoms of schizophrenia (Honer et al., 2012) and high- versus standard-dose risperidone for established schizophrenia (Claus et al., 1992). Based on the findings, the report came to the conclusion that high doses of a (non-clozapine) SGA medication should not be used instead of standard doses for treatment-resistant schizophrenia.

The notion that doses of olanzapine above the licensed maximum may be beneficial for treatment-resistant psychosis has been around for a while (Sheitman et al., 1997; Mountjoy et al., 1999). Several clinical trials have tested the efficacy of high-dose olanzapine against standard doses of clozapine for TRS, and most of these (Conley et al., 1998; Tollefson et al., 2001; Bitter et al., 2004; Meltzer et al., 2008) have reported equivalent efficacy, although not all (Kumra et al., 2008). One meta-analysis of randomized studies comparing clozapine with olanzapine for TRS found no significant differences in efficacy (Asenjo Lobos et al., 2010), while another (Souza et al., 2013) found clozapine to be superior in terms of improvement of positive and negative symptoms. Souza et al. (2013) concluded that, while the most robust evidence for efficacy in TRS supported clozapine, olanzapine, particularly in higher dosage, was a treatment option to be considered.

While prescription of antipsychotic medication above the maximum licensed dose is frequent in clinical practice (Paton et al., 2008; Howes et al., 2012), the consensus statement on high-dose antipsychotic medication by the Royal College of Psychiatrists (2014) concluded that, overall, there was no convincing evidence that antipsychotic dosage higher than the maximum licensed dose is more effective than standard dosage for the treatment of resistant schizophrenia. It concluded that, if such a regimen were to be initiated, it should be as an individual therapeutic trial. Treatment review should consider whether there had been a clinically significant improvement in the target symptoms and weigh any such benefit against emergent and potential adverse effects before deciding whether the high-dose strategy should continue or be adjusted. If continued, there should be appropriate monitoring of side effects given the increased risk with high dose.

Combined antipsychotics (antipsychotic polypharmacy)

As with high-dose antipsychotic prescribing, there is a lack of robust evidence for the efficacy of combined antipsychotic medication (Barnes and Paton, 2011; Ballon and Stroup, 2013). A meta-analysis of 16 relevant studies by Galling et al. (2017) found that antipsychotic augmentation with an SGA medication was superior to continuing monotherapy for total symptoms, but this only applied to open-label and low-quality trials and was not the case in double-blind and high-quality studies. Negative symptoms improved more with augmentation, but only in those studies augmenting with aripiprazole. Thus, high-quality trials generally failed to find symptom improvement and treatment response with augmentation of clozapine or non-clozapine antipsychotic medication with a second antipsychotic.

Prescribing more than one antipsychotic medication for a patient may have a number of adverse consequences. Such a strategy is known to increase the risk of a high-dose prescription (Paton et al., 2008; López de Torre et al., 2012) and drug–drug interactions. It is also associated with a greater global side effect burden, as well as an increased risk of extrapyramidal symptoms, hyperprolactinaemia, sexual dysfunction, hypersalivation, sedation, cognitive impairment, and diabetes (Gallego et al., 2012; Fleischhacker and Uchida, 2014). There is also a greater risk of poor adherence with a more complex drug regimen.

Despite the lack of efficacy found in trials and the potential adverse effects, it remains hard to argue that a combination of antipsychotic medications would never have a reasonable risk–benefit balance for a particular patient with TRS (Lerner et al., 2004; Pandurangi and Dalkilic, 2008). However, Pandurangi and Dalkilic (2008) concluded that the evidence was not sufficient to support the routine use of SGA polypharmacy to treat positive or negative symptoms, 'even as the fourth or fifth step in a treatment algorithm for acute or chronic schizophrenia'.

Augmentation strategies

The augmentation of continuing antipsychotic medication with other medications such as antidepressants, mood stabilizers, and benzodiazepines is commonly tried in clinical practice for treatment-resistant illness prior to the initiation of clozapine (Thompson et al., 2016), but the outcome is often disappointing. Studies of such augmentation have been criticized for their small sample sizes and lack of a rigorous methodology, and the data on efficacy and safety are often only short term (Sinclair and Adams, 2014; Correll et al., 2017a). Critically, while such augmentation strategies may be used in clinical practice to target particular symptoms, the participants in trials may not have been selected for the relevant clinical indication. Further, potential pharmacokinetic issues are rarely addressed. Thus far, no pharmacological combination has warranted approval for TRS as a licensed indication.

Valproate

The evidence supporting valproate as an add-on treatment for people with schizophrenia on continuing antipsychotic medication remains uncertain. Tseng et al. (2016) reported a meta-analysis of studies comparing the treatment effect of antipsychotic medication augmented with valproate with antipsychotic medication with or without placebo in people with schizophrenia or schizoaffective disorder. While valproate augmentation showed significantly more improvement in total psychopathology in open trials, this was not the case in randomized controlled trials (RCTs). Further, improvement was found in short-term (<4 weeks) but not longer-term (≥4 weeks) studies.

Another meta-analysis (Zheng et al., 2017) examined data from studies comparing clozapine augmentation with anticonvulsant agents, including sodium valproate, with clozapine alone. Sodium valproate augmentation was associated with a significant reduction in total Positive And Negative Syndrome Scale (PANSS) score compared with clozapine monotherapy but was not associated with a significant difference when study-defined response was used as the outcome.

In practice, adjunctive valproate is commonly prescribed for the treatment of persistent aggression in TRS. Valproate has been found to have benefit in cases of poor impulsivity with certain personality disorders (Huband et al., 2010), but the evidence in schizophrenia is limited. Wang et al. (2016) concluded that the findings of relevant open RCTs in schizophrenia suggested that, in addition to some efficacy in relation to overall clinical response, augmentation with valproate might have some benefit for specific symptoms such as excitement and aggression. However, if adjunctive valproate is considered for impulsive aggression in schizophrenia, Citrome and Volavka (2011) advise that it only be administered as an individual trial with close monitoring of the benefits as well as safety and tolerability.

If prescribing for a female patient, weighing the risks and benefits of adding valproate should take account of the serious teratogenic potential of valproate, which is dose-related (Tomson et al., 2011; Tomson and Battino, 2012; Campbell et al., 2014), and the national guideline recommendations to avoid prescribing valproate for women of childbearing age (NICE, 2014; Goodwin et al., 2016). If adding valproate to clozapine medication, clinicians should be aware of the potentially increased risk of neutropenia with this combination (Malik et al., 2018).

Lithium

There is no RCT evidence that lithium on its own is an effective treatment for schizophrenia (Leucht et al., 2015). A meta-analysis of studies comparing augmentation of antipsychotic medication with lithium with antipsychotic medication alone in people with schizophrenia or related disorders proved inclusive (Leucht et al., 2004). While more of the patients receiving lithium augmentation were classified as responders, this superiority was not consistent across different response thresholds and, when those patients with prominent affective symptoms were excluded from the analysis, any significant advantage of lithium augmentation was lost. Considering TRS, a meta-analysis of a range of augmentation strategies found no evidence that lithium augmentation of clozapine was superior to clozapine monotherapy (Li et al., 2016). Further, no improvement was seen in forensic patients with TRS when lithium was added as an adjunctive treatment to antipsychotic medication in a 4-week, single-blind, randomized trial (Collins et al., 1991).

Over the years, guideline recommendations, expert opinion, and the findings of a few trials have suggested that adding lithium to antipsychotic medication, including clozapine, may have a place in the treatment of affective symptoms, excitement, aggression, or agitation in people with schizophrenia (Lehman et al., 2004; Lerner et al., 1988; Small et al., 2003; Kontaxakis et al., 2005). However, the evidence for efficacy is thin (Atre-Vaidya and Taylor, 1989; Keck et al., 1996; Correll et al., 2017b). Whether a therapeutic trial of adjunctive lithium would ever be worth considering for a patient with resistant schizophrenia who exhibited persistent affective symptoms, particularly signs of excited behaviour, remains uncertain (Citrome, 2009).

Lamotrigine

As an add-on treatment to non-clozapine antipsychotic medication for patients with residual psychotic symptoms of schizophrenia, the anticonvulsant lamotrigine lacks any convincing evidence for efficacy (Goff et al., 2007). The potential value of lamotrigine as an adjunctive treatment for clozapine-resistant schizophrenia also remains equivocal. A meta-analysis of five studies testing lamotrigine for clozapine-resistant schizophrenia reported benefit for both positive and negative symptoms. The proportion of responders (defined as ≥20% reduction in total PANSS/Brief Psychiatric Rating Scale [BPRS] score) was 41% for lamotrigine versus 10% for placebo (Tiihonen et al., 2009b). However, with removal of one outlier study (Zoccali et al., 2007), lamotrigine was no longer superior to placebo in meta-analyses (Porcelli et al., 2012; Sommer et al., 2012). No benefit was found for lamotrigine augmentation on symptoms or cognitive function in a sample of patients with partial response to clozapine (Vayisoğlu et al., 2013). Further, a meta-analysis of six relevant studies showed only a trend towards reduction of residual positive and negative symptoms (Veerman et al., 2014).

Topiramate

A trend for a positive effect of topiramate, another anticonvulsant medication, on positive and negative symptom scores in schizophrenia that emerged from a meta-analysis of three relevant RCTs disappeared after removal of an outlier study (Sommer et al., 2012). Nevertheless, in subsequent meta-analyses of larger numbers of RCTs, the medication has shown more promise (Zheng et al., 2016; Okuyama et al., 2016). A meta-analysis of 12 RCTs comparing topiramate with placebo or antipsychotic medication alone in people with schizophrenia (Okuyama et al., 2016) found topiramate augmentation to be superior for improving positive, negative, and overall symptoms. However, given the methodological limitations of the studies included, the investigators concluded that the findings could not be applied to 'daily clinical practice'.

Other augmentation strategies

Correll et al., (2017a) conducted an overview of meta-analyses of RCTs comparing the efficacy of add-on medication to antipsychotic treatment with placebo or antipsychotic monotherapy in people with schizophrenia. The data analysed concerned 42 different psychotropic medications, including antidepressants, lamotrigine, selective serotonin-3-receptor antagonists (such as ondansetron and granisetron), oestrogen activity (sex hormones and oxytocin), minocycline, lithium, modafinil, and topiramate. Thirty-seven of the adjunctive strategies were tested with any antipsychotic medication. While in several cases meta-analysis had found significant superiority for the combination, issues regarding study quality, including risk of bias, led Correll et al., (2017a) to conclude that none of these strategies had consistent supporting evidence for use in unselected patients with schizophrenia. None of the five strategies tested with clozapine showed superiority in terms of improvement in total psychopathology. This finding is in line with a review by Muscatello et al., (2014) of studies of augmentation strategies in patients with treatment-refractory schizophrenia treated with clozapine as well as the results of a meta-analysis of relevant studies by Sommer et al., (2012), which concluded that there was currently no replicated evidence that any pharmacological augmentation strategy was an effective treatment for total, positive, or negative symptoms in patients treated with clozapine.

There is no evidence of antipsychotic efficacy with benzodiazepines and, while they may be worth considering for very short-term sedation of acutely agitated patients, they are not appropriate as a medium- to long-term augmentation strategy (Dold et al., 2013). Adjunctive antidepressants may be considered for the treatment of comorbid depressive or persistent negative symptoms, although for the latter any benefit is likely to be modest (Singh et al., 2010; Helfer et al., 2016; Barnes et al., 2016). Promising results for adjunctive electroconvulsive therapy (ECT) in decreasing psychopathology scores in patients with TRS, particularly clozapine-resistant illness, needs further validation (Pawełczyk et al., 2014; Petrides et al., 2015; Kim et al., 2017; Grover et al., 2017). The most common side effects are transient retrograde and anterograde amnesia, headaches, and nausea.

Summary

The use of non-clozapine antipsychotic polypharmacy and high-dose antipsychotic medication for TRS is not supported by the evidence (Miyamoto et al., 2014). For schizophrenia that has shown an insufficient response despite continuing non-clozapine antipsychotic medication, augmentation strategies cannot be considered as alternatives to clozapine in terms of potential efficacy, particularly with regard to positive symptoms, but may be worthwhile to tackle clinically significant target symptoms. In practice, augmentation and combination strategies should be prescribed as individual trials, being closely monitored for effectiveness and adverse effects, and should only be continued if there is evident benefit that outweighs any risks or safety concerns.

REFERENCES

Agid, O., Arenovich, T, Sajeev, G., et al. (2011). An algorithm-based approach to first-episode schizophrenia, response rates over 3 prospective antipsychotic trials with a retrospective data analysis. *J Clin Psychiatry*, 72, 1439–44.

Asenjo Lobos, C., Komossa, K., Rummel-Kluge, C., et al. (2010). Clozapine versus other atypical antipsychotics for schizophrenia. *Cochrane Database of Systematic Reviews*, CD006633.

Atre-Vaidya, N., Taylor, M. A. (1989). Effectiveness of lithium in schizophrenia: do we really have an answer? *J Clin Psychiatry*, 50, 170–3.

Ballon, J., Stroup, T. S. (2013). Polypharmacy for schizophrenia. *Curr Opin Psychiatry*, 26, 208.

Barnes, T. R. E., Paton, C. (2011). Antipsychotic polypharmacy in schizophrenia: benefits and risks. *CNS Drugs*, 25, 383–99.

Barnes, T. R. E., Leeson, V. C., Paton, C., et al. (2016). Antidepressant Controlled Trial For Negative Symptoms In Schizophrenia (ACTIONS): a double-blind, placebo-controlled, randomised clinical trial. *Health Technol Assess*, 20, 1–46.

Bitter, I., Dossenbach, M. R., Brook, S., et al. Olanzapine HGCK Study Group. (2004). Olanzapine versus clozapine in treatment-resistant or treatment-intolerant schizophrenia. *Prog Neuropsychopharmacol Biol Psychiatry*, 28, 173–80.

Campbell, E., Kennedy, F., Russell, A., et al. (2014). Malformation risks of antiepileptic drug monotherapies in pregnancy: updated results from the UK and Ireland Epilepsy and Pregnancy Registers. *J Neurol Neurosurg Psychiatry*, 85, 1029–34.

Canadian Agency for Drugs and Technologies in Health. (2011). *Optimal use recommendations for atypical antipsychotics: combination and high-dose treatment strategies in adolescents and adults with schizophrenia*. Volume 1, Issue 1C. Ottawa: Canadian Agency for Drugs and Technologies in Health.

Citrome, L., (2009). Adjunctive lithium and anticonvulsants for the treatment of schizophrenia: what is the evidence? *Expert Rev Neurother*, 9, 55–71.

Citrome, L., Volavka, J. (2011). Pharmacological management of acute and persistent aggression in forensic psychiatry settings. *CNS Drugs*, 25, 1009–21.

Claus, A., Bollen, J., DeCuyper, H., et al. (1992). Risperidone versus haloperidol in the treatment of chronic schizophrenic inpatients: a multicentre double-blind comparative study. *Acta Psychiatr Scand*, 85, 295–305.

Collins, P. J., Larkin, E. P., Shubsachs, A. P. (1991). Lithium carbonate in chronic schizophrenia—a brief trial of lithium carbonate added to neuroleptics for treatment of resistant schizophrenic patients. *Acta Psychiatr Scand*, 84, 150–4.

Conley, R. R., Tamminga, C. A., Bartko, J. J., et al. (1998). Olanzapine compared with chlorpromazine in treatment-resistant schizophrenia. *Am J Psychiatry*, 155, 914–20.

Correll, C. U., Rubio, J. M., Inczedy-Farkas, G., Birnbaum, M. L., Kane, J. M., Leucht, S. (2017a). Efficacy of 42 pharmacologic cotreatment strategies added to antipsychotic monotherapy in schizophrenia: systematic overview and quality appraisal of the meta-analytic evidence. *JAMA Psychiatry*, 74, 675–84.

Correll, C. U., Yu, X., Xiang, Y., Kane, J. M., Masand, P. (2017b). Biological treatment of acute agitation or aggression with schizophrenia or bipolar disorder in the inpatient setting. *Ann Clin Psychiatry*, 29, 92–107.

Davis, J. M., Chen, N. (2004). Dose response and dose equivalence of antipsychotics. *J Clin Psychopharmacol*, 24, 192–208.

Dold, M., Leucht, S. (2014). Pharmacotherapy of treatment-resistant schizophrenia: a clinical perspective. *Evid Based Ment Health*, 17, 33–7.

Dold, M., Li, C., Gillies, D., Leucht, S. (2013). Benzodiazepine augmentation of antipsychotic drugs in schizophrenia: a meta-analysis and Cochrane review of randomized controlled trials. *Eur Neuropsychopharmacol*, 23, 1023–33.

Dold, M., Fugger, G., Aigner, M., Lanzenberger, R., Kasper, S. (2015). Dose escalation of antipsychotic drugs in schizophrenia: a meta-analysis of randomized controlled trials. *Schizophr Res*, 166, 187–93.

Fleischhacker, W. W., Uchida, H. (2014). Critical review of antipsychotic polypharmacy in the treatment of schizophrenia. *Int J Neuropsychopharmacol*, 17, 1083–93.

Frogley, C., Taylor, D., Dickens, G., et al. (2012). A systematic review of the evidence of clozapine's anti-aggressive effects. *Int J Neuropsychopharmacol*, 15, 1351–71.

Gallego, J. A., Nielsen, J., De Hert, M., Kane, J. M., Correll, C. U. (2012). Safety and tolerability of antipsychotic polypharmacy. *Expert Opin Drug Saf*, 11, 527–42.

Galling, B., Roldán, A., Hagi, K., et al. (2017). Antipsychotic augmentation vs. monotherapy in schizophrenia: systematic review, meta-analysis and meta-regression analysis. *World Psychiatry*, 16, 77–89.

Gardner, D. M., Murphy, A. L., O'Donnell, H., Centorrino, F., Baldessarini, R. J. (2010). International consensus study of antipsychotic dosing. *Am J Psychiatry*, 167, 686–93.

Goff, D. C., Keefe, R., Citrome, L., et al. (2007). Lamotrigine as add-on therapy in schizophrenia: results of 2 placebo-controlled trials. *J Clin Psychopharmacol*, 27, 582–9.

Goodwin, G. M., Haddad, P. M., Ferrier, I. N., et al. (2016). Evidence-based guidelines for treating bipolar disorder: revised third edition recommendations from the British Association for Psychopharmacology. *J Psychopharmacol*, 30, 495–553.

CHAPTER 9

Grover, S., Chakrabarti, S., Hazari, N., Avasthi, A. (2017). Effectiveness of electroconvulsive therapy in patients with treatment resistant schizophrenia: a retrospective study. *Psychiatry Res,* 249, 349–53.

Hasan, A., Falkai, P., Wobrock, T., et al. (2012). World Federation of Societies of Biological Psychiatry (WFSBP) Task Force on Treatment Guidelines for Schizophrenia. World Federation of Societies of Biological Psychiatry (WFSBP) Guidelines for Biological Treatment of Schizophrenia, part 1: update 2012 on the acute treatment of schizophrenia and the management of treatment resistance. *World J Biol Psychiatry,* 13, 318–78.

Helfer, B., Leucht, S., Rothe, P. H., et al (2015). Increasing antipsychotic dose for non response in schizophrenia. *Cochrane Database Syst Rev,*10, CD011883.

Helfer, B., Samara, M. T., Huhn, M., et al. (2016). Efficacy and safety of antidepressants added to antipsychotics for schizophrenia: a systematic review and meta-analysis. *Am J Psychiatry,* 173, 876–86.

Honer, W. G., MacEwan, G. W., Gendron, A., et al. STACK Study Group. (2012). A randomized, double-blind, placebo-controlled study of the safety and tolerability of high-dose quetiapine in patients with persistent symptoms of schizophrenia or schizoaffective disorder. *J Clin Psychiatry,* 73, 13–20.

Howes, O. D., Vergunst, F., Gee S., McGuire P., Kapur S., Taylor D. (2012). Adherence to treatment guidelines in clinical practice: study of antipsychotic treatment prior to clozapine initiation. *Br J Psychiatry,* 201, 481–5.

Huband, N., Ferriter, M., Nathan, R., Jones, H. (2010). Antiepileptics for aggression and associated impulsivity. *Cochrane Database Syst Rev,* 17(2), CD003499.

Kane, J., Honigfeld, G., Singer, J., Meltzer, H. (1988). Clozapine for the treatment-resistant schizophrenic: a double-blind comparison with chlorpromazine. *Arch Gen Psychiatry,* 45, 789–96.

Keck, P. E. Jr., McElroy, S. L., Strakowski, S. M. (1996). New developments in the pharmacologic treatment of schizoaffective disorder. *J Clin Psychiatry,* 57 (Suppl. 9), 41–8.

Kim, H. S., Kim, S. H., Lee, N. Y., et al. (2017). Effectiveness of electroconvulsive therapy augmentation on clozapine-resistant schizophrenia. *Psychiatry Investig,* 14, 58–62.

Kontaxakis, V. P., Ferentinos, P. P., Havaki-Kontaxaki, B. J., Roukas, D. K. (2005). Randomized controlled augmentation trials in clozapine-resistant schizophrenic patients: a critical review. *Eur Psychiatry,* 20, 409–15.

Kumra, S., Kranzler, H., Gerbino-Rosen, G., et al. (2008). Clozapine and 'high-dose' olanzapine in refractory early-onset schizophrenia: a 12-week randomized and double-blind comparison. *Biol Psychiatry,* 63, 524–9.

Lally, J., Ajnakina, O., Di Forti, M., et al. (2016). Two distinct patterns of treatment resistance: clinical predictors of treatment resistance in first-episode schizophrenia spectrum psychoses. *Psychol Med,* 46, 3231–40.

Lambert, T. J. (2007). Switching antipsychotic therapy: what to expect and clinical strategies for improving therapeutic outcomes. *J Clin Psychiatry,* 68 (Suppl. 6), 10–13.

Lehman, A. F., Lieberman, J. A., Dixon, L. B., et al. American Psychiatric Association; Steering Committee on Practice Guidelines. (2004). Practice guideline for the treatment of patients with schizophrenia, second edition. *Am J Psychiatry,* 161 (2 Suppl.), 1–56.

Lerner, V., Libov, I., Kotler, M., Strous, R. D. (2004). Combination of 'atypical' antipsychotic medication in the management of treatment-resistant schizophrenia and schizoaffective disorder. Prog Neuropsychopharmacol Biol Psychiatry, 28, 89–98.

Lerner, Y., Mintzer, Y., Schestatzky, M. (1988). Lithium combined with haloperidol in schizophrenic patients. Br J Psychiatry, 153, 359–62.

Leucht, S., Kissling, W., McGrath, J. (2004). Lithium for schizophrenia revisited: a systematic review and meta-analysis of randomized controlled trials. J Clin Psychiatry, 65, 177–86.

Leucht, S., Cipriani, A., Spineli, L., et al. (2013). Comparative efficacy and tolerability of 15 antipsychotic drugs in schizophrenia: a multiple-treatments meta-analysis. Lancet, 382, 951–62.

Leucht, S., Helfer, B., Dold, M., Kissling, W., McGrath, J. J. (2015). Lithium for schizophrenia. Cochrane Database Syst Rev, 10, CD003834.

Li, Y. Y., Zhang, Y. S., Wang, J., Li, K. Q., Wang, H. Y. (2016). Optimal treatment strategies of clozapine for refractory schizophrenia. Zhongguo Yi Xue Ke Xue Yuan Xue Bao, 38, 666–78.

López de Torre, A., Lertxundi, U., Hernández, R., Medrano, J. (2012). Antipsychotic polypharmacy: a needle in a haystack? Gen Hosp Psychiatry, 34, 423–32.

Malik, S., Lally, J., Ajnakina, O., et al. (2018). Sodium valproate and clozapine induced neutropenia. A case control study using register data. Schizophr Res, 195, 267–73.

McEvoy, J. P., Lieberman, J. A., Stroup, T. S., et al. (2006). Effectiveness of clozapine, quetiapine and risperidone in patients with chronic schizophrenia who failed prior atypical antipsychotic treatment. Am J Psychiatry, 153, 600–10.

Meltzer, H. Y., Alphs, L., Green, A. I., et al. (2003). Clozapine treatment for suicidality in schizophrenia: International Suicide Prevention Trial (InterSePT). Arch Gen Psychiatry, 60, 82–91.

Meltzer, H. Y., Bobo, W. V., Roy, A., et al. (2008). A randomized, double-blind comparison of clozapine and high-dose olanzapine in treatment-resistant patients with schizophrenia. J Clin Psychiatry, 69, 274–85.

Miyamoto, S., Jarskog, L. F., Fleischhacker, W. W. (2014). New therapeutic approaches for treatment-resistant schizophrenia: a look to the future. J Psychiatr Res, 58, 1–6.

Mountjoy, C. Q., Baldacchino, A. M., Stubbs, J. H. (1999). British experience with high-dose olanzapine for treatment-refractory schizophrenia. Am J Psychiatry, 156, 158–9.

Muscatello, M. R., Bruno, A., De Fazio, P., et al. (2014). Augmentation strategies in partial responder and/or treatment-resistant schizophrenia patients treated with clozapine. Expert Opin Pharmacother, 15(16), 2329–45.

NICE. (2014). Bipolar Disorder: assessment and management. Clinical guideline 185.

Okuyama, Y., Oya, K., Matsunaga, S., Kishi, T., Iwata, N. (2016). Efficacy and tolerability of topiramate-augmentation therapy for schizophrenia: a systematic review and meta-analysis of randomized controlled trials. Neuropsychiatr Dis Treat, 12, 3221–36.

Pandurangi, A. K., Dalkilic, A. (2008). Polypharmacy with second-generation antipsychotics: a review of evidence. J Psychiatr Pract, 14, 345–67.

Paton, C., Barnes, T. R. E., Cavanagh, M-R., Taylor, D., on behalf of the POMH-UK project team. (2008). High-dose and combination antipsychotic prescribing in acute adult wards in the UK; the challenges posed by PRN. Br J Psychiatry, 192, 435–9.

Pawełczyk, T., Kołodziej-Kowalska, E., Pawełczyk, A., Rabe-Jabłońska, J. (2014). Augmentation of antipsychotics with electroconvulsive therapy in treatment-resistant schizophrenia patients with dominant negative symptoms: a pilot study of effectiveness. *Neuropsychobiology*, 70, 158–64.

Petrides, G., Malur, C., Braga, R. J., et al. (2015). Electroconvulsive therapy augmentation in clozapine-resistant schizophrenia: a prospective, randomized study. *Am J Psychiatry*, 172, 52–8.

Porcelli, S., Balzarro, B., Serretti, A. (2012). Clozapine resistance: augmentation strategies. *Eur Neuropsychopharmacol*, 22, 165–82.

Ringbäck Weitoft, G., Berglund, M., et al. (2014). Mortality, attempted suicide, re-hospitalisation and prescription refill for clozapine and other antipsychotics in Sweden—a register-based study. *Pharmacoepidemiol Drug Saf*, 23, 290–8.

Royal College of Psychiatrists. (2014). *Consensus Statement on High-Dose Antipsychotic Medication*. College Report CR190.

Samara, M., Leucht, S. (2016). Treatment strategies in case of non-response in schizophrenia: meta-analytical assessments of increasing the antipsychotic dose and switching the antipsychotic drug versus continuation of the same antipsychotic dose and drug, Poster T252. 5th Biennial Schizophrenia International Research Society Conference, Florence, Italy, 2016.

Samara, M. T., Dold, M., Gianatsi, M., et al. (2016). Efficacy, acceptability, and tolerability of antipsychotics in treatment-resistant schizophrenia: a network meta-analysis. *JAMA Psychiatry*, 73, 199–210.

Sheitman, B. B., Lindgren, J. C., Early, J., Sved, M. (1997). High-dose olanzapine for treatment-refractory schizophrenia. *Am J Psychiatry*, 154, 1626.

Sinclair, D., Adams, C. E. (2014). Treatment resistant schizophrenia: a comprehensive survey of randomised controlled trials. *BMC Psychiatry*, 14, 253.

Singh, S. P., Singh, V., Kar, N., et al. (2010). Efficacy of antidepressants in treating the negative symptoms of chronic schizophrenia: meta-analysis. *Br J Psychiatry*, 197, 174–9.

Siskind, D., McCartney, L., Goldschlager, R., Kisely, S. (2016). Clozapine v. first- and second-generation antipsychotics in treatment-refractory schizophrenia: systematic review and meta-analysis. *Br J Psychiatry*, 209, 385–92.

Small, J. G., Klapper, M. H., Malloy, F. W., Steadman, T. M. (2003). Tolerability and efficacy of clozapine combined with lithium in schizophrenia and schizoaffective disorder. *J Clin Psychopharmacol*, 23, 223–8.

Sommer, I. E., Begemann, M. J., Temmerman, A., Leucht, S. (2012). Pharmacological augmentation strategies for schizophrenia patients with insufficient response to clozapine: a quantitative literature review. *Schizophr Bull*, 38, 1003–11.

Souza, J. S., Kayo, M., Tassell, I., et al. (2013). Efficacy of olanzapine in comparison with clozapine for treatment-resistant schizophrenia: evidence from a systematic review and meta-analyses. *CNS Spectr*, 18, 82–9.

Stauffer, V. L., Case, M., Kinon, B. J., et al. (2011). Early response to antipsychotic therapy as a clinical marker of subsequent response in the treatment of patients with first-episode psychosis. *Psychiatry Res*, 187, 42–8.

Takeuchi, H., Kantor, N., Uchida, H., Suzuki, T., Remington, G. (2017). Immediate vs gradual discontinuation in antipsychotic switching: a systematic review and meta-analysis. *Schizophr Bull*, 43, 862–71.

Thompson, J. V., Clark, J. M., Legge, S. E., et al. (2016). Antipsychotic polypharmacy and augmentation strategies prior to clozapine initiation: a historical cohort study of 310 adults with treatment-resistant schizophrenic disorders. *J Psychopharmacol*, 30, 436–43.

Tiihonen, J., Lönnqvist, J., Wahlbeck, K., et al. (2009a). 11-year follow-up of mortality in patients with schizophrenia: a population-based cohort study (FIN11 study). *Lancet*, 374, 620–7.

Tiihonen, J., Wahlbeck, K., Kiviniemi, V. (2009b). The efficacy of lamotrigine in clozapine-resistant schizophrenia: a systematic review and meta-analysis. *Schizophr Res*, 109, 10–14.

Tollefson, G. D., Birkett, M. A., Kiesler, G. M., Wood, A. J.; Lilly Resistant Schizophrenia Study Group. (2001). Double-blind comparison of olanzapine versus clozapine in schizophrenic patients clinically eligible for treatment with clozapine. *Biol Psychiatry*, 49, 52–63.

Tomson, T., Battino, D. (2012). Teratogenic effects of antiepileptic drugs. *Lancet Neurol*, 11, 803–13.

Tomson, T., Battino, D., Bonizzoni, E., et al.; EURAP study group. (2011). Dose-dependent risk of malformations with antiepileptic drugs: an analysis of data from the EURAP epilepsy and pregnancy registry. *Lancet Neurol*, 10, 609–17.

Tseng, P. T., Chen, Y. W., Chung, W., et al. (2016). Significant effect of valproate augmentation therapy in patients with schizophrenia: a meta-analysis study. *Medicine (Baltimore)*, 95, e2475.

Vayısoğlu, S., Anıl Yağcıoğlu, A. E., Yağcıoğlu, S., et al. (2013). Lamotrigine augmentation in patients with schizophrenia who show partial response to clozapine treatment. *Schizophr Res*, 143, 207–14.

Veerman, S. R., Schulte, P. F., Begemann, M. J., Engelsbel, F., de Haan, L. (2014). Clozapine augmented with glutamate modulators in refractory schizophrenia: a review and metaanalysis. *Pharmacopsychiatry*, 47, 185–94.

Wang, Y., Xia, J., Helfer, B., Li, C., Leucht, S. (2016). Valproate for schizophrenia. *Cochrane Database Syst Rev*, 11, CD004028.

Weiden, P. J. (2006). Switching in the era of atypical antipsychotics. An updated review. *Postgrad Med*, Spec No, 27–44.

Yoshimura, B., Yada, Y., So, R., Takaki, M., Yamada, N. (2017). The critical treatment window of clozapine in treatment-resistant schizophrenia: secondary analysis of an observational study. *Psychiatry Res*, 250, 65–70

Zheng, W., Xiang, Y. T., Xiang, Y. Q., et al. (2016). Efficacy and safety of adjunctive topiramate for schizophrenia: a meta-analysis of randomized controlled trials. *Acta Psychiatr Scand*, 134, 385–98.

Zheng, W., Xiang, Y. T., Yang, X. H., Xiang, Y. Q., de Leon, J. (2017). Clozapine augmentation with antiepileptic drugs for treatment-resistant schizophrenia: a meta-analysis of randomized controlled trials. *J Clin Psychiatry*, 78, e498–e505.

Zoccali, R., Muscatello, M. R., Bruno, A., et al. (2007). The effect of lamotrigine augmentation of clozapine in a sample of treatment-resistant schizophrenic patients: a double-blind, placebo-controlled study. *Schizophr Res*, 93, 109–16.

CHAPTER 9

Psychosis and the family: the role of family interventions

Juliana Onwumere and Elizabeth Kuipers

KEY POINTS

- The development of a psychotic illness exerts a significant impact on the affected individual but also affects their family and social networks, often leading to a substantial burden on carers.

- Although psychotic conditions are severe mental health problems, they are treatable, and family care and support play an important role in helping to achieve better recovery outcomes.

- High expressed emotion within families is associated with poorer outcomes in patients with psychotic disorders, and is linked to particular illness beliefs in carers.

- Positive affect and warmth in carers is associated with reduced relapse rates in people with psychotic disorders.

- Family interventions are evidence based talking therapies designed to help people living with psychosis and their families. They aim to improve understanding of psychosis and its related problems. It focuses on supporting families in developing skills in positive communication, problem-solving, coping, and identifying appropriate support pathways.

- Family interventions are included in several treatment and best practice guidance for psychosis. Systematic reviews and data syntheses confirm that family interventions significantly reduce relapse and hospitalisation rates in patient groups and positively impact carer outcomes, including reducing levels of burden. The interventions have large effect sizes, with proven cost effective and scalability in routine services.

Background

Despite experiencing high levels of social isolation, a majority of individuals with psychosis will receive a substantial degree of their care and support from informal carers. These carers are mainly close relatives such as parents, partners, siblings, and adult offspring. Assuming an informal caregiving role will often be a long-term undertaking, which partly reflects the complexity of the problems and their course. Few carers report having made an active decision or being given a choice in taking on their caregiving role. Nevertheless, support from informal carers is widely recognized as being invaluable and making a significant contribution to ensuring positive patient outcomes, including accessing the right care and support during the initial phase.

In England, the concealed financial value of caregiver support has been estimated at 1.24 billion pounds per annum (The Schizophrenia Commission, 2012), with approximately 5.5% of carers giving up paid employment to undertake their unpaid caregiving role (Mangalore and Knapp, 2007). The current literature suggests that people with psychosis who have family support, when compared to those without, tend to experience significantly fewer relapses in their illness and hospitalizations (Norman et al., 2005). Family support is also predictive of improved life expectancy. In a 10-year follow-up of first-onset psychosis patients, a 90% reduction in mortality rates was recorded for those who had family involvement at initial onset (Revier et al., 2015).

Impact of caregiving role

Psychosis and the caregiving role can have an adverse impact on the overall health and positive wellbeing of carers. Historically, this impact has mainly been described and measured using the concept of 'burden'. A large number of carers report experiencing carer burden. Stress- and mood-related disorders are common in all caregiver groups when compared to the general population (Smith et al., 2014). In a review of data obtained from the English Adult Psychiatric Morbidity Survey 2007, the results confirmed significantly higher rates of common mental disorders in those with caregiving responsibilities. The negative impact on mental health was notable for those completing 10 hours or more care each week, with a twofold increase in those caring at 20 hours or more per week (Smith et al., 2014). In psychosis carers, 30–40% experience clinical depression and psychological distress (Hamaie et al., 2016; Hayes et al., 2015) and a similar proportion (i.e. 44%) report post-traumatic stress symptoms (Kingston et al., 2016). Reports of psychological distress in carers can be particularly high during the first episode (Jansen et al., 2015).

Carers can report feeling exhausted and 'burnt out' in their role in the same way and at similar levels to those observed in professional psychiatric staff groups. This clinical presentation is already evident in carers of first-episode groups even in the first few months and years following initial onset of difficulties (Onwumere et al., 2017a). Similar to the relatives for whom they provide care, informal carers are socially isolated. Hayes et al. (2015) reported that carers of people with psychosis, when compared to non-caregiving peers, were approximately 10 times more isolated. Carers of people with psychosis are also known to report greater isolation and lower support than carers of other equivalent long-term physical health conditions (e.g. brain injury, heart illnesses) (Magliano et al., 2005).

As part of their role, carers are often exposed to a broad range of confusing, problematic, and, at times, antisocial behaviours, including violence (Onwumere et al., 2014). Recent data suggest that approximately 30% of carers can report being the target of patient-initiated violence during the preceding year (Kageyama et al., 2016). Families also report experiencing high levels of stigma, which can impact on their access to services and support. Reports of self-blame, confusion, loss, and bewilderment are commonplace, particularly at first onset (McCann et al., 2011). The physical health of carers is also impacted by their caregiving role. These include notable disturbances in carer reports of sleep and an overall poorer quality of life (Hayes et al., 2015; Smith et al., 2018).

Although there is a smaller body of research, the experience of caregiving can also be associated with positive experiences and satisfaction (Kulhara et al., 2012). Positive caregiving experiences include, for some carers, improvements in the quality of the relationship with the person for whom they care, alongside an improved sense of self, self-esteem, and an awareness of their inner strengths and life priorities (Chen and Greenberg, 2004). Positive experiences can exist in parallel with negative experiences, but they are independent, with different influencing factors and associated outcomes (Onwumere et al., 2008).

Impact of caregiving: implications for patient and carer outcomes

Family carers who are negatively impacted by their roles can also experience difficulties in their coping abilities and the relationship with the person for whom they provide care. For example, carers reporting high levels of burden and psychological distress are also more likely to engage in less adaptive styles of coping (i.e. coping through avoidance, just hoping things will go away) (Onwumere et al., 2011b). In addition, these carers are also more likely to have caregiving relationships characterized by high expressed emotion (EE) (Jansen et al., 2014). EE has been defined as a quantifiable measure of family climate and the quality of family interactions and relationships. It is measured across five key dimensions: criticism, hostility, emotional overinvolvement, warmth, and positive comments. High EE relationships are those characterized by carers reporting high levels of criticism, hostility, and/or emotional overinvolvement (EOI) towards the person for whom they care (Vaughn and Leff, 1976). Conversely, low EE ratings reflect carers who did not score above threshold on any of these three scales. Illustrative EE speech comments are reported in Table 10.1.

High EE caregiving relationships are predictive of less favourable recovery outcomes for people with psychosis, which include a greater number and longer duration of hospital admissions (Marom et al., 2005) and shorter time to relapse (Koutra et al., 2015). To illustrate, data from two widely cited meta-analytic reviews of EE outcome studies indicate that individuals with psychosis in high EE caregiving relationships are at least twice as likely to experience a relapse in their psychosis compared to low EE groups (Bebbington and Kuipers, 1994). The high EE patient relapse link is particularly the case for individuals in high EE relationships characterized by high levels of carer criticism (Cechnicki et al., 2013).

Exposure to high EE relationships can impact on overall brain functioning and individual symptoms. Rylands et al. (2011) completed functional magnetic resonance assessments on individuals with psychosis to assess exposure to familial high EE. The results highlighted a differential pattern of brain activation in areas

Table 10.1 Expressed emotion illustrative speech comments

Expressed emotion component	Illustrative quote
Criticism	It really *irritates* me how we can never sit through a family meal without Simon talking to those voices
Hostility	I'd rather just leave him (in hospital)… There comes a point when you've just got to put your foot down
Emotional overinvolvement	We don't like leaving him on his own … ever'
Warmth	I prefer her to go out on her own to give her confidence
Positive comments	Mike is an excellent sportsman.

concerned with the processing of aversive social information (e.g. rostral anterior cingulate, middle superior frontal gyrus) following exposure to high EE stimuli.

Illness beliefs

High EE relationships are important not only because of their predictive links with relapse but because they are distinguishable by different underlying illness beliefs reported by carers (Barrowclough and Hooley, 2003), even at first onset (Dominguez-Marinez et al., 2017). High EE relationships characterized by criticism and hostility are associated with carers who are less inclined to appraise their relative's problems as being part of an illness but instead view their problems as something they (i.e. the relative with psychosis) are responsible for (i.e. are doing deliberately, and could stop *if* they wanted to). Further, reports of carer shame have been linked to carer expressions of criticism/hostility. Conversely, overinvolved caregiving relationships are associated more with carers who blame themselves for their relative's problems, feel guilty about and perceive their relative as having no control over their problems (Barrowclough and Hooley, 2003). These carers are also more likely to experience feelings of shame and guilt (Cherry et al., 2017).

The patient perspective in caregiving relationships

People with psychosis are sensitive to the behaviours and actions of others and can accurately perceive negative affect from caregivers (Onwumere et al., 2009). Furthermore, their perceptions of carer affect can impact on their functioning and overall outcomes (Tomlinson et al., 2013) and have a greater impact than actual carer affect (Tompson et al., 1995).

Positive family relationships

The importance of positivity in familial styles of communications, behaviour interactions, and overall family atmosphere has been increasingly recognized and documented in the mental health literature, particularly in terms of its implications for reducing the risk of developing psychosis in children and young people presenting with high familial risk for psychosis (Tienari et al., 2004) or subclinical prodromal symptoms (O'Brien et al., 2006). Expressions of warmth also form an important feature of the EE index and can impact on illness course and family outcomes (Bebbington and Kuipers, 1994), particularly in some ethnic groups (Singh et al., 2013). In a review of 65 first-episode psychosis families, Lee et al. (2014) found that patients were less likely to relapse during a 6- and 12-month follow-up period when they perceived greater levels of positive affect from carers or when carers were rated highly for warmth.

Family interventions

The different strands of research on carer burden, family relationships, and their predictive links with patient outcomes and, more recently, patient perceptions of carer affect, have independently fed into the development of evidence-based family approaches to working with people with psychosis. The provision of this kind of family work has been included in several treatment guidelines across the globe, including Canada, Europe, Australia, and the USA (Norman et al., 2017; NICE, 2014; Galletly et al., 2016; Kreyenbuhl et al., 2010). The National Institute for Health and Care Excellence (NICE) for England, Wales, and Northern Ireland treatment guidelines recommends the provision of family interventions to all families who are in close contact with service users with psychosis. The duration of interventions should last for between 3 months and 1 year, with a minimum of 10 sessions. These recommendations have been in existence for several years, having first been included in the early 2000s (NICE, 2003; 2009; 2014).

We know that the needs of families, where a relative has psychosis, are often complex and will differ from one family to the next. Nevertheless, the current literature suggests that families have a need for emotional support alongside advice and information that can help to facilitate a better individualized understanding of the illness, and how best to cope with presenting symptoms and crises (Askey et al., 2009).

There is some variation in the composition and delivery of evidence-based family interventions. They can differ on variables such as the length of an intervention, location of where sessions are held (e.g. home versus clinic), whether the patient is included in none, some, or all of the sessions, and whether sessions are delivered with a single family or multiple groups of families in one sitting (Kuipers et al., 2002; McFarlane, 2002). They do, however, share several core features. These include an underlying stress vulnerability conceptualization of psychosis onset and maintenance, a focus on the issues currently affecting the family, and reducing future risk of patient relapse. The interventions are offered, explicitly, because a family member has psychosis and not because of any theories pertaining to an underlying family dysfunction. In addition, all family members are enlisted as partners in care and recovery outcomes. The interventions, which are professionally led, are offered as an adjunct to medication and other treatments (Box 10.1).

Box 10.1 Key features of evidence-based family interventions

- Use a stress vulnerability model of psychosis
- Use a normalizing approach to family responses and reactions to caregiving
- Therapists are open and transparent
- Therapists have a non-blaming and positive attitude to families
- Use a collaborative approach to working with and alongside the family
- Family members are approached and enlisted as positive therapeutic agents
- Needs and the strengths of the family are explicitly acknowledged
- Focus on current problems
- Professionally led
- Forms part of a wider package of care

Family interventions are designed to promote changes in cognitive, behavioural, and emotional domains, and incorporate key therapeutic strategies based on providing information about psychosis (psychoeducation), facilitating skills in positive communication, problem-solving and adaptive coping, emotional support, and stress management (Gracio et al., 2016a; Kuipers et al., 2002). As a minimum, family intervention sessions are usually held on a fortnightly basis and typically two therapists will be involved in delivering the intervention (Kuipers et al., 2002).

Family perspectives on their experience of engaging in family interventions and the perceived key components of change have been encouraging. In a qualitative review of 12 patients with psychosis and 14 relatives who had engaged with family interventions, the perceived benefits of the interventions were varied but included an improved understanding of the illness, family communication, and problem-solving, and recognition of early indicators of relapse (Nilsen et al., 2016). Likewise, as part of a qualitative investigation of 10 participants who had received family interventions, Rapsey et al. (2015) reported that the interventions facilitated a greater understanding about psychosis and provided a safe space to discuss difficult and sensitive issues and explore unhelpful ways of relating to one another.

The evidence base for family interventions

There exists a long and robust evidence base in support of the efficacy and effectiveness of family interventions in psychosis, with more than 50 randomized controlled trials (RCTs) (Sin et al., 2017; Pharoah et al., 2010). Data from one of the largest Cochrane reviews of 53 RCTs confirmed that family interventions in schizophrenia led to significant reductions in rates of patient relapse and hospitalization, and reductions in high EE ratings (Pharoah et al., 2010). The review findings, which were consistent with other studies, also attest to family interventions making a significant and positive impact on social functioning in patients (Pfammatter et al., 2006) and in reducing their levels of medication non-compliance

(Pharoah et al., 2010; Pilling et al., 2002). Family interventions have proved effective in recent-onset psychosis groups (e.g. Claxton et al., 2017; Ma et al., 2017; Onwumere et al., 2011a) and those deemed at high risk of developing psychosis (O'Brien et al., 2014). In their recent meta-analytic review of family interventions in early psychosis populations, Claxton et al. (2017) reported that family interventions significantly reduced patient relapse and improved their functioning at treatment end. Carers also benefited, with significant improvements in levels of carer burden and positive wellbeing. In addition, following a course of family interventions, carers rated high EE at baseline were more likely to be reclassified as low EE (Claxton et al., 2017). In a review of carer outcomes following family interventions in early psychosis, Ma et al. (2017) also confirmed the superiority of family interventions, when compared to standard treatment, for improving carer burden, and identified that these positive changes also improve over time. The authors reported a large effect size for reductions in burden ($g = -0.97$, confidence interval [CI] $= -1.49$ to -0.46).

The impact of interventions is not limited to patient outcomes only. Family interventions can also yield positive results for informal carers, as illustrated by significant reductions in preintervention levels of burden (Giron et al., 2010) and increases in positive caregiving appraisals and readiness to continue in their caregiving role (Berglund et al., 2003). In addition to generating favourable postintervention outcomes for patient and carers, family interventions have proven cost-efficacy (NICE, 2009) and are scalable and effective when applied in routine services (Ruggeri et al., 2015). Longer term follow-up studies also offer support for their efficacy. Recent data from a 14-year follow-up study of family interventions in China highlighted improved social functioning in patients' work capability and medication compliance in those receiving family interventions compared to the control group (Ran et al., 2016).

Family intervention provision

Despite the evidence base, to date, one of the biggest issues related to family interventions is its poor implementation and the patchy access to it recorded across different regions. This can range between 0% in some areas to 53% in others (Ince et al., 2016; Prytys et al., 2011). Several reasons have been proposed to explain the poor access figures. These include workforce issues such as lack of training programs and adequately skilled staff, insufficient supervision, competing time demands, and service priorities for practitioners (Onwumere et al., 2016). Further explanations have also included pessimistic beliefs reported by staff about the need for and benefits of family interventions in helping to alleviate the presenting difficulties of families, and difficulties in successfully engaging families (Prytys et al., 2011).

Although evidence-based family interventions are recommended in several treatment guidelines, it is increasingly acknowledged that not all families will want or indeed require the full intervention or be in a position or area to access it (Onwumere et al., 2016; Gracio et al., 2016b; Cohen et al., 2008). As raised earlier, we know that families typically present with a range of needs, which vary in the level of expert input required to facilitate positive and meaningful changes. Limiting full and longer duration interventions to a much smaller group of families (e.g. families where a patient may frequently relapse), who are likely to present with the highest levels of clinical need and complexity, appears sensible in an era of much reduced resources (Onwumere et al., 2016).

Cohen et al. (2008) represented one of the first groups to propose a triage-based approach to family interventions, whereby the focus remained on delivering the least clinically intensive type of family work able to yield positive family outcomes and minimize carer distress. The comprehensive evidence-based family interventions were positioned at the highest level, with preceding levels comprising intermittent family work, brief education sessions and crisis work, and a family-friendly and inclusive service.

Case illustration: Michael and Sylvia*

The Marden family provides an illustration of key therapeutic activities typically observed in family interventions in psychosis. For the reader, it is important to note that, in family interventions, the different aspects of the work (e.g. problem-solving, psychoeducation, facilitating positive communication) will often overlap within individual sessions and these are therefore not delivered in isolation or in a linear fashion. For example, to address issues of psychoeducation will invariably require work on communication styles and may also involve problem-solving and emotional processing.

Michael is a young, white, British-born man in his early thirties with an approximate 11-year history of psychosis and diagnosis of schizophrenia. His first-onset of psychosis occurred during his second year at university where he was studying for a science undergraduate degree. Michael was admitted to a local psychiatric inpatient facility for 5 months, under a section of the Mental Health Act 1983 (as amended in 2007). Over the course of his mental health difficulties, Michael has had several inpatient admissions, with most being under section and with the longest admission lasting for 11 months. During his hospital admissions, the acute and distressing nature of his presenting symptoms tend to improve to a sufficient degree to support a discharge but, following discharge and a return to community-based living, there has often been a slow and repeated pattern of deterioration in his functioning alongside disengagement from services and prescribed pharmacological treatments.

Michael experienced a complex set of persecutory delusional beliefs that were held with high conviction. The beliefs related to ongoing worries about being

* To preserve anonymity, the following is a composite case using pseudonyms and no identifiable details.

subject to a 'surveillance order' and having his belongings interfered with by an underground, powerful, global, and secret government-like organization. During periods of relapse, the interference beliefs also extended towards his food and drinks being tampered with and the people close to him (e.g. family, mental health staff) being 'got at'. According to Michael, he was being targeted by the organization, their ultimate intention being to kill him, because of the organization's incorrect intelligence that he witnessed an event that he was not meant to and which could reveal their existence to others. The all-powerful and all-knowing organization was able to influence the actions of many others and thus he was typically suspicious and mistrusting of those around him. He experienced high levels of distress and preoccupation with his beliefs, and fluctuating auditory verbal hallucinatory experiences that were attributed to the organization. He struggled with different aspects of his social functioning that included maintaining regular patterns of self-care. He believed that the organization was capable of monitoring him wherever he went and, during periods of relapse and crises, he often found it difficult to bathe or use the toilets owing to concerns about surveillance. Michael was supported by a community mental health team that included having an assigned care coordinator, who was a community psychiatric nurse. He recently had a relapse (6 months ago) for which he was hospitalized for 10 weeks.

Michael lived at home with his mother Sylvia, who was in her mid-60s and retired. Sylvia previously worked in an administrator role but resigned from her job almost 9 years ago to care for her son. He had no siblings and had never had contact with his father. Sylvia undertook all of the household chores, including Michael's laundry and making the family meals. She also tried to make sure that her son attended his appointments with the team. Sylvia experienced high blood pressure, for which her general practitioner had highlighted a need for Sylvia to explore pathways for addressing any impacting stressors.

Following a routine offer of family interventions that was presented to the family during a recent care plan review meeting, Michael and Sylvia had both agreed to meet for family sessions with two family intervention therapists resident in the community team. Although offers of family intervention had been made previously, both Michael and his mother had either declined or Michael had declined with reports that it was not the right time. Until recently, offers of individual psychology therapy had also previously been declined by Michael, but he was currently on a waiting list for cognitive behavioural therapy for psychosis (see Chapter 11).

As part of the ongoing therapy engagement process, it was agreed with Michael and Sylvia that the family sessions would take place within the family home. Sessions would be held at midday or later to support Michael's likely attendance and engagement. During sessions, in agreement with the family, the television and other background entertainment devices were switched off (e.g. radio) to minimize obvious distractions that would invariably occur were they to be on. The family were seen for a total of 13 sessions over 8 months. Sessions were always an hour long with no less than a minimum of a fortnight between scheduled

CHAPTER 10

meetings. Although the family were offered a minimum of 10 sessions and were initially in agreement about having the family meetings, the therapists agreed with the family to build in a review of the sessions after the third appointment and, depending on the outcome of those discussions, build in further reviews at three-session intervals. This was done to help the family to establish a greater sense of control over the intervention and how it would and could develop. As part of the process to ensure that both therapists actively engaged with both family members, it was planned that one therapist would always lead on engagement with one family member each session, while the second therapist engaged with the other family member and they would alternate this focus at every meeting. This approach helped to minimize the risk of either Michael or Sylvia feeling that only one therapist understood their perspective. The process of facilitating engagement was also supported through the therapist being empathic, validating, and using active listening techniques (e.g. summarizing what they had heard and checking in with each family member whether they had understood things correctly). The therapist also sought feedback from each family member at the end of each session to address and pick up on any misunderstandings. The therapists were both clinical psychologists with training in family interventions.

In the initial family session the therapists commenced by talking through an agenda, and providing an overview (and reiteration of pre-engagement conversations they had held with Michael and Sylvia) about what family interventions were and how they (i.e. the therapists) usually worked in family meetings. This involved a discussion about the therapists not wanting to make things worse for the family and the acknowledgement that they had plenty of time, if the family wanted to, to work together on issues of importance to them both. The therapists also acknowledged the time and effort that Sylvia and Michael had both made to ensure the first meeting happened. The communication ground rules were then explicitly introduced by the therapists (i.e. one person to talk at a time, direct speech, where possible, between family members, and the plan that both Michael and Sylvia would have equal talking time). The therapists made a point of noting that these communication styles might already be something the family do anyway, but emphasized that it was something the therapists found helpful when having family meetings and they would support the family throughout the meetings to observe these styles, with a recognition that it might mean the therapists interrupting individuals from time to time to keep us all on track. The remainder of the first session was then used to get a brief idea of the important areas (i.e. therapy goals) that Michael and Sylvia would like to work on and in which they wished to see an improvement.

The question about therapy goals was first directed at Michael. He explained that his goals for the intervention were to have fewer arguments with his mother because these often left him feeling emotional and tired afterwards. He reported that he had begun to think recently that he would prefer for his mother and himself not to speak to one another rather than to argue as often as they did. He did not think that his mother understood very much about his everyday challenges because, if she did, he did not think they would argue. During the process of Michael reporting on his therapy goals, Sylvia needed some therapist support (and in subsequent sessions) to avoid her tendency to interrupt Michael as he talked and provide a response. She was asked if she could 'hold on' to her important comments for a little bit and reassured that she would have her turn shortly to talk, but for now it was important to hear what Michael was saying. For Sylvia's goals, she explained that she wanted Michael to listen to her and take her instructions about helping him to get better. She felt that he did not want to improve because, if he did, he would listen to her. Sylvia explained that she had always found it difficult to understand why Michael seemed to make progress in hospital but slow down when he came out of hospital. Although she was aware of his mental health problems, she could never quite understand why he could not help more with some household tasks. The therapists commented that identifying areas of their relationship that they would like to develop and improve upon was a shared goal and a helpful place to start. It was also noted that Sylvia appeared to have a need to understand more about the type of difficulties that Michael experienced, which also overlapped with his goal of wanting his mother to understand more about the things with which he had to cope. The therapists acknowledged that, at any point over the course of their meetings, Michael and Sylvia might also identify further therapy goals and that it would be okay to bring those to the meetings.

Thus, in line with the agreed therapy goals, the next few sessions focused in more detail on how the family were communicating with each other, identifying the common issues about which they often found themselves arguing, and problem-solving key areas. It was soon clear from both their accounts that what tended to act as a constant trigger to some of the discord in their relationship was the lack of a break (i.e. space) that either family member had from one another and the absence of positive events and interactions in their relationship. Michael's beliefs about surveillance had meant that he restricted a lot of his movements about where he would go and at what times he would feel comfortable leaving the home. Thus, Michael and his mother were spending most parts of the day at home with one another and their conversations were often related to things about which they were unhappy or disappointed. The therapists highlighted how *any* relationship would be under strain under similar circumstances and when there was a lack of positive exchanges and shared interests. To support the focus on improving communication styles, the family agreed on a 'homework' activity where they identified one small pleasant and achievable task they could do together that they *both* liked and they could feed back how it went in the sessions. Through discussion they initially agreed on eating a sandwich in their garden, which was something that they both enjoyed doing many years ago as both were keen gardeners. They were able to complete the homework task over a period of three sessions and then added further activities to their pleasant task list that included watching a nature programme together and planting some new flowers, which they both enjoyed doing.

Not dissimilar to many other carers, it was clear that Sylvia had become increasingly socially isolated over the years that she had spent caring for Michael.

She had gradually lost touch with most of the small circle of friends that she had prior to the onset of her son's mental health problems. She had used to attend a dance fitness class, swim, and be part of a work-based choir. Sylvia expressed that she was reluctant to attend things because she had insufficient time to complete the household chores and support her son with his medication. The importance of looking after herself and paying attention to her own wellbeing was discussed by the therapists, with Michael's contribution sought. The therapists discussed the importance of Sylvia aiming to have something (e.g. an activity) of her own on which she could focus. The idea of meeting up with other parents and carers in similar roles was also discussed. Michael was able to share with his mother that he felt that she should have some time on her own in the week because of all the work that she did, and he was concerned that she often looked sad and tired, which were comments that also precipitated some tears from Sylvia. Michael and Sylvia were supported to problem-solve one thing they might need to modify in their current timetable to facilitate Sylvia spending some time away from the family home for one morning a week. It was agreed that, for this change to be facilitated, there would need to be alternative arrangements for the preparation of Michael's breakfast. Hitherto, Sylvia would prepare a cooked egg breakfast for her son. As part of the problem-solving discussion, Michael had identified a solution where he could have a boiled egg sandwich or just have cereal and could try leading on organizing his own breakfast for that one morning a week.

The therapists learnt that Sylvia did not really speak to anyone (e.g. friends, peers) about her experiences. There was a mental health carers group coffee morning that was running at a local carer resource centre that Sylvia agreed to visit to see what it was like. Carer support groups can provide an important source of information, emotional support, and an exchange of helpful coping strategies to manage the everyday common problems that families typically have to face. They can also provide a safe and containing platform where carers are able to be open about the broad range of emotions (e.g. anger, guilt, frustration, annoyance, despair, fear) they can experience in the caregiving role and how they feel about the person for whom they are caring (Kuipers et al., 2002). In groups, carers' feelings and experiences can be normalized, validated, and understood without explanation and a feeling of being judged (Onwumere et al., 2017b). The therapists were also able to discuss with the family the parallel need for a little bit of extra team 'support' (i.e. help) for Michael to have some regular time off from being at home all of the time too. Following the successes of spending some time in the garden, Michael agreed to meeting with a support worker from his community team for just one afternoon (1.5 hours) per week. They would arrange to go for a coffee to review different horticultural events and resources that he might wish to attend.

In terms of additional triggers to their arguments, Michael and Sylvia both noted that issues concerning medication (specifically, Sylvia's ongoing concern and associated strategies for prompting Michael to take his medication at exactly the same time each day) were areas that often led to arguments. The family were encouraged to share with each other what they were finding difficult and why.

Michael explained that he found his mother's monitoring of him and his behaviour too much and it often left him wondering about her intentions which, in turn, confused him and negatively impacted his mood. He recognized that he became more irritable and unsure of things. Sylvia was able to verbalize her concerns about Michael's history of relapsing and going into hospital and the subsequent guilt that she always felt and a feeling that she would be blamed by others (e.g. clinical staff) for allowing it to happen. Hence, it was important to avoid a relapse and actively do what she could to ensure that Michael was doing all the right things with his medication. She was concerned about how the illness had developed and how Michael would fare at a stage when she would no longer be around to offer support.

Both reported that this had been the first time they had heard the comments from one another and that it had been helpful to listen and understand the other's perspective. The therapists were able to identify Sylvia's concern and love for Michael that ran underneath her medication-monitoring behaviours and their shared goal to avoid making things worse with how Michael was feeling. Time was given to problem-solving how Michael was able to have (and feel that he had) more control about taking his medication and to feel less monitored by his mother. This included session work where Michael discussed with Sylvia the times that suited him for taking his nighttime medication. A homework exercise was agreed where Michael would take the lead on taking his medication at the agreed time, and for them both to feed back on how the exercise left them feeling. Although it was not listed as one of their original therapy aims, the therapists agreed with the family that it might also be helpful to spend some time developing a family relapse prevention plan. The concerns and anxieties about a relapse were normalized.

In line with their agreed therapy aims, the information sharing (psychoeducation) aspect of the intervention was a useful tool to support Michael and Sylvia's understanding of psychosis and how it specifically related to their first-hand (lived) experience. As part of this work, Michael was able to talk directly with his mother about some of his experiences, particularly the beliefs that could preoccupy much of his thinking time and how they could interfere with the attention he was able to give to other things, including sleep. Michael was able to report that there were also times that he was able to cope with his experiences much better than others (or times when the beliefs were less bothersome), and these included time spent in the garden and times when he did not feel upset from having an argument. The psychoeducation sessions, which commenced from session 5, also focused on other symptom experiences (e.g. negative symptoms, hallucinations, thinking difficulties), causal explanations, groups affected by psychosis, and recovery. The process ended with the agreed plan to develop a family relapse prevention plan. Time was given to supporting Michael and Sylvia to identify and discuss the early indicators of relapse that they both noticed and what helpful strategies they could both use to access appropriate support. They had both agreed to share a copy of the plan with Michael's care coordinator. Sylvia commented that, although she had been caring for her son for over a decade, she was not aware of many of the experiences that he reported during the psychoeducation sections of the intervention. She reported that Michael's therapy goals for wanting to reduce their arguments (and improve the quality of their relationship) made greater sense to her now.

By the end of the intervention, Sylvia had progressed to spending two after-noons and one morning a week outside the family home. This time included at-tending a carer group and engaging in a yoga and swimming class. She was able to report that she had enjoyed the family meetings and, although it had been difficult at times, she was pleased she kept going with the sessions. She found the carer group supportive and had recently exchanged a contact number with another group member who was also a mother. Michael and his mother both felt the overall quality of their relationship had improved; they reported having sig-nificantly fewer arguments. When asked what they felt had led to these changes, they both reported that they felt more listened to by the other person. Since the early sessions, they had continued to enjoy their weekly 'pleasant activity' slot, which the therapists felt had positively influenced the expressed warmth between Michael and Sylvia and what they had to talk about.

Supporting families in the future

As we look towards future developments in working with families who are sup-porting relatives with mental health difficulties, digital innovations and advance-ments in web-based interventions are increasingly gaining attention (Onwumere and Kuipers, 2017; www.futurelearn.com/courses/caring-psychosis-schizophrenia). Such approaches have the potential to reach a greater number of individuals in need, in a cost- and time-effective manner. They also offer flexible styles of engagement with interventions; for example, being able to access the required support while at home. Thus far, the evidence in support of the acceptability and impact of web-based interventions has been positive. Rotondi et al. (2010) piloted online provision of multi-family work for 31 people with psychosis and their carers. The authors reported significant improvements in levels of illness understanding in participants.

It is widely acknowledged that much of the work on family approaches in psych-osis that have been investigated have been interventions and initiatives led by pro-fessional mental health staff. There is, however, a small but growing body of work that has begun to look at the importance and impact of family support approaches facilitated by carer peers. Dixon et al. (2011) investigated outcomes from a peer-led 12-week family education programme for carers of people with mental health problems as part of a randomized intervention. In a sample of 318 relatives, signifi-cant improvements in problem-solving, coping, illness understanding, and feelings of empowerment were recorded in those participating in the intervention.

Conclusion

The onset of a severe mental health problem can be life-changing not only for the individual person receiving the diagnosis but also for their family and support network. Although services and care provision have clearly developed and improved over the years, it still remains the case that families can find themselves feeling overwhelmed, confused, bewildered, frightened, guilty, and angry about their circumstances and how best to address the many challenges to which they are suddenly exposed. This process is likely to be complicated by experiences of stigma, including self-stigma and loss. In recognition of these challenges, approaches to upskilling families, offering support, and facilitating a better and more informed understanding of the problems remains an important component of service and treatment guidelines. The evidence base attesting to the efficacy of family approaches when working with psychosis continues to underpin the justification for their inclusion in treatment guidelines. Further work is required on how best to ensure greater equitable access to evidence-based and family-inclusive interventions in psychosis to improve outcomes and facilitate family recovery.

REFERENCES

Askey, R., Holmshaw, J., Gamble, C., Gray, R. (2009). What do carers of people with psychosis need from mental health services? Exploring the views of carers, service users and professionals. *J Fam Ther*, 31, 310–31.

Barrowclough, C., Hooley, J. M. (2003). Attributions and expressed emotion: a review. *Clin Psychol Rev*, 23(6), 849–80.

Bebbington, P., Kuipers, L. (1994). The clinical utility of expressed emotion in schizophrenia. *Acta Psych Scand Suppl*, 382, 46–53.

Berglund, N., Vahlne, J. O., Edman, A. (2003). Family intervention in schizophrenia—impact on family burden and attitude. *Soc Psychiatry Psychiatric Epidemiol*, 38(3), 116–21.

Cechnicki, A., Bielanska, A., Hanuszkiewicz, I., Daren, A. (2013). The predictive validity of expressed emotions (EE) in schizophrenia. A 20-year prospective study. *J Psychiatric Res*, 47(2), 208–14.

Chen, F.P., Greenberg, J.S. (2004). A positive aspect of caregiving: the influence of social support on caregiving gains for family members of relatives with schizophrenia. *Community Ment Health J*, 40(5), 423–35.

Cherry, M. G., Taylor, P. J., Brown, S. L., Rigby, J. W., Sellwood, W. (2017). Guilt, shame and expressed emotion in carers of people with long term mental health difficulties: a systematic review. *Psychiatry Res*, 249, 139–51.

Claxton, M., Onwumere, J., Fornells-Ambrojo, M. (2017). Do family interventions improve outcomes in early psychosis? A systematic review and meta-analysis. *Frontiers Psychol*, 8, 371.

Cohen, A. N., Glynn, S. M., Murray-Swank, A. B., et al. (2008). The family forum: directions for the implementation of family psychoeducation for severe mental illness. *Psychiatr Serv*, 59(1), 40–8.

Dixon, L. B., Lucksted, A., Medoff, D. R., et al. (2011). Outcomes of a randomized study of a peer-taught family-to-family education program for mental illness. *Psychiatr Serv*, 62(6), 591–7.

Dominguez-Marinez, T., Medina-Pradas, C., Kwapil, T. R., Barrantes-Vidal, N. (2017). Relatives expressed emotion, distress and attributions in clinical high risk and recent onset psychosis. *Psychiatr Res*, 247, 323–9.

Galletly, C., Castle, D., Dark, F., et al. (2016). Royal Australian and New Zealand College of Psychiatrists clinical practice guidelines for the management of schizophrenia and related disorders. *Aust N Z J Psychiatry*, 50(5), 410–72.

Giron, M., Fernandez-Yanez, A., Mana-Alvarenga, S., Molina-Habas, A., Nolasco, A., Gomez-Beneyto, M. (2010). Efficacy and effectiveness of individual family intervention on social and clinical functioning and family burden in severe schizophrenia: a 2-year randomized controlled study. *Psychol Med*, 40(1), 73–84.

Gracio, J., Goncalves-Pereira M., Leff, J. (2016a). Key elements of a family intervention for schizophrenia. A qualitative analysis of an RCT. *Fam Process*, 57, 100–12.

Gracio, J., Goncalves-Pereira M., Leff, J. (2016b). What do we know about family interventions for psychosis at the process level? A systematic review. *Fam Process*, 55(1), 79–90.

Hamaie, Y., Ohmuro, N., Katsura, M., et al. (2016). Criticism and depression among the caregivers of at risk mental state and first episode psychosis patients. *PLoS One*, 11, e0149875.

Hayes, L., Hawthorne, G., Farhall, J., O'Hanlon, B., Harvey, C. (2015). Quality of life and social isolation among caregivers of adults with schizophrenia: policy and outcomes. *Comm Mental Health J*, 51(5), 591–7.

Ince, P., Haddock, G., Tai, S. (2016). A systematic review of the implementation of recommended psychological interventions for schizophrenia: rates, barriers, and improvement strategies. *Psychol Psychother. Theory Research and Practice*, 89, 324–50.

Jansen, J. E., Lysaker, P. H., Harder, S., et al. (2014). Positive and negative caregiver experiences in first-episode psychosis: emotional overinvolvement, wellbeing and metacognition. *Psychol Psychother. Theory Research and Practice*, 87(3), 298–310.

Jansen, J.E., Gleeson, J., Cotton, S. (2015). Towards a better understanding of caregiver distress in early psychosis: a systematic review of the psychological factors involved. *Clin Psychol Rev*, 35, 56–66.

Kageyama, M., Solomon, P., Kita, S., et al. (2016). Factors related to physical violence experienced by parents of persons in Japan. *Psychiatry Res*, 243, 439–45.

Kingston, C., Onwumere, J., Keen, N., Ruffell, T., Kuipers, E. (2016). Post traumatic symptoms in caregivers of people with psychosis and associations with caregiving experiences. *J Trauma Dissoc*, 17(3), 307–21.

Koutra, K., Triliva, S., Roumeliotaki, T., et al. (2015). Impaired family functioning in psychosis and its relevance to relapse: a two year follow up study. *Compr Psychiatry*, 62, 1–12.

Kuipers, E., Leff, J., Lam, D. (2002). *Family Work for Schizophrenia: a practical guide*, 2nd edn. London: Gaskell.

Kulhara, P., Kate, N., Grover, S., Nehra, R. (2012). Positive aspects of caregiving in schizophrenia: a review. *World J Psychiatry*, 2(3), 43–8.

Kreyenbuhl, J., Buchanan, R. W., Dickerson, F. B., Dixon, L. B. (2010). The schizophrenia Patient Outcomes Research Team (PORT): updated treatment recommendations 2009. *Schizophr Bull*, 36(1), 94–103.

Lee, G., Barrowclough, C., Lobban, F. (2014). Positive affect in the family environment protects against relapse in first-episode psychosis. *Soc Psychiatry Psychiatric Epidemiol*, 49(3), 367–76.

Ma, C. F., Chien, W. T., Bressington, D. T. (2017). Family intervention for caregivers of people with recent-onset psychosis: A systematic review and meta-analysis. *Early Intervention in Psychiatry*, 1–26. doi: 10.1111/eip.12494.

Magliano, L., Fiorillo, A., De Rosa, C., Malangone, C., Maj, M.; National Mental Health Working Group (2005). Family burden in long-term diseases: a comparative study in schizophrenia vs. physical disorders. *Soc Sci Med*, 61(2), 313–22.

Mangalore, R., Knapp, M. (2007). Cost of schizophrenia in England. *J Mental Health Policy Econ*, 109, 23–41.

Marom, S., Munitz, H., Jones, P. B., Weizman, A., Hermesh, H. (2005). Expressed emotion: relevance to rehospitalisation in schizophrenia over 7 years. *Schizophr Bull*, 31(3), 751–8.

McCann, T. V., Lubman, D. I., Clark, E. (2011). First-time primary caregivers' experience of caring for young adults with first-episode psychosis. *Schizophr Bull*, 37(2), 381–8.

McFarlane, W. R. (2002). *Multifamily Groups in the Treatment of Severe Psychiatric Disorders*. New York and London: Guildford Press.

National Institute for Health and Care Excellence. (NICE) (2003). *NICE Guidelines for Psychological Treatment in Schizophrenia*. London: Gaskell Press.

National Institute for Health and Care Excellence. (NICE) (2009). Schizophrenia—Core Interventions in the Treatment and Management of Schizophrenia in Adults in Primary and Secondary. Clinical Guideline 82. London: NICE.

National Institute for Health and Care Excellence. (2014). *Psychosis and Schizophrenia in Adults: treatment and management*. Clinical Guideline 178. London: NICE.

Nilsen, L., Frich, J. C., Friis, S., Norheim, I., Rossberg, J. I. (2016). Participants' perceived benefits of family intervention following a first episode of psychosis: a qualitative study. *Early Intervention in Psychiatry*, 10(2), 152–9.

Norman, R., Lecomte, T., Addington, D., Anderson, E. (2017). CPA treatment guidelines on psychosocial treatment of schizophrenia in adults. *Can J Psychiatry/La Revue Canadienne de Psychiatrie*, 62, 617–23.

Norman, R. M. G., Malla, A. K., Manchanda, R., Harricharan, R., Takhar, J., Northcott, S. (2005). Social support and three-year symptom and admission outcomes for first episode psychosis. *Schizophr Res*, 80, 227–34.

O'Brien, M. P., Gordon, J. L., Bearden, C. E., Lopez, S. R., Kopelowicz, A., Cannon, T. D. (2006). Positive family environment predicts improvement in symptoms and social functioning among adolescents at imminent risk for onset of psychosis. *Schizophr Res*, 81(2–3), 269–75.

O'Brien, M. P., Miklowitz, D. J., Candan, K. A., et al. (2014). A randomized trial of family focused therapy with populations at clinical high risk for psychosis: effects on interactional behavior. *J Consulting Clin Psychol*, 82(1), 90–101.

Onwumere, J., Kuipers, E. (2017). Does the internet have a role in helping the families of people with psychosis? *Psychiatr Serv*, 68(4), 419–20.

Onwumere, J., Kuipers, E., Bebbington, P., et al. (2008). Care-giving and illness beliefs in the course of psychotic illness. *Can J Psychiatry*, 53(7), 460–8.

Onwumere, J., Kuipers, E., Bebbington, P., et al. (2009). Patient perceptions of caregiver criticism in psychosis: links with patient and caregiver functioning. *J Nervous Mental Dis*, 197, 85–91.

Onwumere, J., Bebbington, P., Kuipers, E. (2011a). Family interventions in early psychosis: specificity and effectiveness. *Epidemiol Psychiatr Sci*, 20(2), 113–19.

Onwumere, J., Kuipers, E., Bebbington, P., et al. (2011b). Coping styles in carers of people with recent and long-term psychosis. *J Nervous Mental Dis*, 199(6), 423–4.

Onwumere, J., Grice, S., Garety, P., et al. (2014). Caregiver reports of patient-initiated violence in psychosis. *Can J Psychiatry*, 59(7), 376–84.

Onwumere, J., Grice, S., Kuipers, E. (2016). Delivering cognitive-behavioural family interventions for schizophrenia. *Aust Psychol*, 51, 52–61.

Onwumere, J., Lotey, G., Schulz, J., et al. (2017a). Burnout in early course psychosis caregivers: the role of illness beliefs and coping styles. *Early Interv Psychiatry*, 11 (3), 237–43.

Onwumere, J., Zhou, Z., Desai, R., Learmonth S., Reynolds, N., Gaughran, F. (2017b). Attending a long-term support group for carers of adults with psychosis: a carer's perspective. *J Psychiatr Intens Care*, 13(2), 93–9.

Pfammatter, M., Junghan, U. M., Brenner, H. D. (2006). Efficacy of psychological therapy in schizophrenia: conclusions from meta-analyses. *Schizophr Bull*, 32 (Suppl. 1), S64–80.

Pharoah, F., Mari, J., Rathbone, J., Wong, W. (2010). Family intervention for schizophrenia. *Cochrane Database Syst Rev*, 12, CD000088.

Pilling, S., Bebbington, P., Kuipers, E., et al. (2002). Psychological treatments in schizophrenia: I. Meta-analysis of family intervention and cognitive behaviour therapy. *Psychol Med*, 32(5), 763–82.

Prytys, M., Garety, P. A., Jolley, S., Onwumere, J., Craig, T. (2011). Implementing the NICE guideline for schizophrenia recommendations for psychological therapies: a qualitative analysis of the attitudes of CMHT staff. *Clin Psychol Psychother*, 18(1), 48–59.

Ran, MS., Chui, CHK., Wong, IY-L., et al. (2016). Family caregivers and outcome of people with schizophrenia in rural china: 14 year follow up study. *Soc Psychiatry Psychiatr Epidemiol*, 51, 513–20.

Rapsey, E.H.S., Burbach, F.R., & Reibstein, J. (2015). Exploring the process of family interventions for psychosis in relation to attachment, attributions and problem-maintaining cycles: an IPA study. *Journal of Family Therapy*, 37: 509–528 doi: 10.1111/1467–6427.12085.

Revier, C. J., Reininghaus, U., Dutta, R., et al. (2015). Ten-year outcomes of first-episode psychoses in the MRC AESOP-10 Study. *J Nerv Mental Dis*, 203(5), 379–86.

Rotondi, A. J., Anderson, C. M., Haas, G. L., et al. (2010). Web-based psychoeducational intervention for persons with schizophrenia and their supporters: one-year outcomes. *Psychiatr Serv*, 61(11), 1099–105.

Ruggeri, M., Bonett, C., Lasalvia, A., et al. (2015). Feasibility and effectiveness of a multi-element psychosocial intervention for first-episode psychosis: results from the cluster-randomized controlled get up piano trial in a catchment area of 10 million inhabitants. *Schizophr Bull*, 41(5), 1192–203.

Rylands, A. J., Mckie, S., Elliot, R., Deakin, J. F. W., Tarrier, N. (2011). A functional magnetic resonance imaging paradigm of expressed emotion in schizophrenia. *J Nerv Mental Dis*, 199, 25–9.

Sin, J., Gillard, S., Spain, D., Cornelius, V., Chen, T. and Henderson, C. (2017). Effectiveness of psychoeducational interventions for family carers of people. *Clinical Psychology Review*, 56, 13–24. doi: https://doi.org/10.1016/j.cpr.2017.05.002.

Singh, S. P., Harley, K., Suhail, K. (2013). Cultural specificity of emotional over involvement: a systematic review. *Schizophr Bull*, 39(2), 449–63.

Smith, L., Onwumere, J., Craig, T., McManus, S., Bebbington, P., Kuipers, E. (2014). Mental and physical illness in caregivers: results from an English national survey sample. *Br J Psychiatry*, 205(3), 197–203.

Smith, L., Onwumere, J., Craig, T & Kuipers, E. (2018). A role for poor sleep in determining distress in caregivers of individuals with early psychosis. *Early Intervention in Psychiatry*. doi: 10.1111/eip.12538.

The Schizophrenia Commission. (2012). *The Abandoned Illness: a report from the Schizophrenia Commission*. London: Rethink Mental Illness.

Tienari, P., Wynne, L. C., Sorri, A., et al. (2004). Genotype–environment interaction in schizophrenia-spectrum disorder—long-term follow-up study of Finnish adoptees. *Br J Psychiatry*, 184, 216–22.

Tomlinson, E., Onwumere, J., Kuipers, E. (2013). Distress and negative experiences of the care-giving relationship in early psychosis—does social cognition play a role? *Early Interv Psychiatry*, 8(3), 253–260.

Tompson, M. C., Goldstein, M. J., Lebell, M. B., Mintz, L. I., Marder, S. R., Mintz, J. (1995). Schizophrenic-patients perceptions of their relatives' attitudes. *Psychiatry Res*, 57, 155–67.

Vaughn, C. E., Leff., J. P. (1976). The measurement of expressed emotion in families of psychiatric patients. *Br J Soc Clin Psychol*, 15(2), 157–65.

Cognitive behaviour therapy for psychosis

Majella Byrne, Suzanne Jolley, and Emmanuelle Peters

KEY POINTS

- Cognitive behaviour therapy for psychosis (CBTp) addresses maladaptive information processing, cognitive biases, and behavioural responses that may lead to and maintain distressing psychotic symptoms.

- CBTp is generally given in addition to pharmacotherapy and not as a replacement for drug treatment, although there is some evidence for a benefit in patients who stop or choose not to take antipsychotic medication.

- The therapist works collaboratively with the patient to develop a formulation of factors that maintain the distress of the psychotic symptoms and their origins.

- Therapy aims to help the patient to modify maladaptive beliefs and unhelpful behavioural responses to reduce the distress and functional impact of symptoms.

- There have been over 50 trials of CBTp, and meta-analyses show benefits for CBTp on a number of outcomes, including psychotic symptom severity and relapse prevention, with moderate effect sizes.

- Meta-analysis of 16 trials specifically in patients with antipsychotic-resistant psychotic symptoms shows a moderate–large benefit of CBTp that persists after therapy ends.

Cognitive behaviour therapy for psychosis

CBTp is based on CBT approaches for emotional disorders, as expounded by Beck in the 1960s, with adaptations for individuals experiencing distressing psychotic symptoms. CBTp is usually offered in addition to pharmacotherapy. The basic CBT model proposes that, in a given situation, a person's emotional, physiological, and behavioural responses to their experiences are driven by appraisals of the meaning of those experiences rather than necessarily the experiences per se. Appraisals are influenced by a person's overarching beliefs ('schema') about themselves, others, and the world, which are formed through their life experiences. Beck proposed that psychopathology resulted from maladaptive information processing or cognitive biases, which lead to distorted and problematic thinking, such as overgeneralizing or drawing a global conclusion from one or more negative experiences (e.g. 'nothing ever goes well for me') or dichotomous thinking, where things are seen in absolutes (e.g. 'if I can't do everything, then I'm totally useless'). Problematic thinking, in turn, leads directly to negative emotions and counterproductive behaviours. The aim of CBT is to identify the psychological processes leading to, and maintaining, the distressing appraisals and problematic responses. Therapy involves developing a shared cognitive behavioural understanding of the difficulties, and finding alternative, less distressing, meanings and new ways of responding to reduce distress and improve functioning.

Cognitive models of psychotic symptoms (Garety et al., 2001; Morrison, 2001; Bentall et al., 2007; Chadwick and Birchwood, 1994) vary in their emphasis on what is appraised, including anomalous perceptions (e.g. hearing a voice), emotional changes, other life events, or any intrusion into awareness, whether external or internal in origin. Models also vary in specifying the kinds of appraisals that are problematic, from external, personal, and threatening (Garety et al., 2001), to culturally unacceptable (Morrison, 2001), to uncontrollable and powerful (Chadwick and Birchwood, 1994). In addition to schema, and the thinking biases typically associated with emotional disorders, distressing appraisals are also influenced by cognitive biases characteristic of psychosis, such as jumping to conclusions and externalizing attributional biases. Once a distressing belief is formed, normal belief maintenance processes, such as searching for confirmatory evidence, come into play. Maladaptive coping behaviours (e.g. using alcohol or drugs) or 'safety behaviours' (e.g. hypervigilance to threat and avoidance of situations or people) are often adopted by people to keep themselves safe, but prevent them from checking out the veracity of their appraisal, thus maintaining conviction and associated distress. CBTp therapists work with people to break these vicious cycles by developing an individually tailored, helpful understanding of their psychotic experiences that identifies triggers, promotes adaptive coping, and addresses unhelpful or negative appraisals. An example formulation of the maintenance of distress from voices is outlined in Fig. 11.1.

Despite Beck publishing a case study of CBTp in 1952, it was not until the 1990s that the first books on the application of CBTp were published (Fowler et al., 1995; Kingdon and Turkington, 1994; Chadwick et al., 1996) and empirically based models of psychosis were developed (Chadwick and Birchwood, 1994; Freeman et al., 2002; Garety et al., 2001; 2007; Morrison, 2001; Bentall et al., 2007). Over the next decade, therapeutic approaches progressed from being generic for schizophrenia/psychosis to focusing on specific symptoms, such as delusions (Freeman et al., 2006; 2008) and voices (Hayward et al., 2012; Meaden et al., 2012), and specific populations and stages of psychosis (French and Morrison, 2004; Van Der Gaag et al., 2013; Gumley and Schwannauer, 2006). More recently, third-wave approaches have developed. These focus on changing how the person relates to distressing experiences, encouraging acceptance of

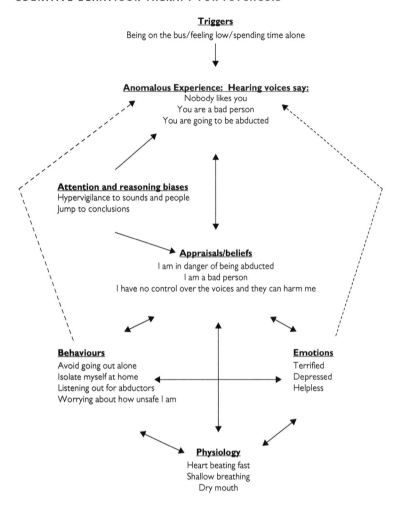

Fig. 11.1 Example of a formulation of persisting voices.

them rather than trying to get rid of them, and working towards the person's values with a view to improving their quality of life, regardless of their experiences (Morris et al., 2013; Wright et al., 2014). Overall, the heterogeneity of presentation in psychosis means that therapy approaches are diverse, with up to 30 books and manuals currently available.

CHAPTER 11

Therapeutic components of cognitive behaviour therapy for psychosis

In line with CBTp models, reframing appraisals and modifying behaviour related to psychotic symptoms are the main mechanisms of change, with the overarching aim of reducing distress and improving functioning and wellbeing. Therapy is collaborative, facilitating active participation from the client, who is seen as an expert in his or her experiences. Therapists discuss psychotic symptoms as human experiences, understandable by normal psychological processes, which make sense in the context of the person's life experiences (Morrison and Barratt, 2010). Change is facilitated by a good therapeutic relationship (Goldsmith et al., 2015) and is based on a shared formulation. Addressing emotional processes is at the heart of CBTp, since all cognitive models identify the important role of emotions in the formation and maintenance of psychotic symptoms (Birchwood, 2003; Freeman and Garety, 2003). Therapy is geared towards the person's personal valued goal(s), with paramount importance being given to maintaining the person's self-esteem, empowering and providing hope, and promoting recovery-orientated values such as attaining a more meaningful and personally fulfilling life (Brabban et al., 2016). A brief description of therapeutic approaches for delusions and hallucinations, respectively, is provided in the sections on 'Cognitive behaviour therapy for delusions' and 'Cognitive behaviour therapy for hallucinations' (for recent overviews see Hunter et al., 2014; Morrison, 2017; Lincoln and Peters, 2018).

Cognitive behaviour therapy for delusions

CBT for delusions is not a 'technical' therapy aimed at 'challenging' delusions. The emphasis is on reducing the dimensions of distress, preoccupation, and impact on functioning, and increasing the patient's sense of control and hope, rather than necessitating conviction change. Outcomes vary, ranging from full conviction change (i.e. the person no longer believes the delusion is true) to 'working within the delusion', where no conviction change is expected but therapy is focused on changing emotional and behavioural sequelae (e.g. the person continues to believe they are being monitored but he or she has discovered that ignoring the persecutor and engaging with valued activities reduces distress and improves mood). Therapeutic work occurs within the context of a shared formulation of the factors maintaining distress and adverse impact, and sometimes of the origins of the belief. The formulation provides the rationale for cognitive and behavioural work, such as making sense of beliefs about the world being a dangerous place owing to developmental adverse experiences, targeting triggers (emotional and/ or situational) and maintenance factors, or changing 'safety behaviours' to test the likelihood and severity of harm. Much of the work is carried out at the 'process' rather than the 'content' level, i.e., changing *how* people think rather than *what* they believe, since people with delusions present with many of the typical Beckian biases found in depression, such as the tendency to dwell on negative rather than neutral or positive material, and anxiety, such as focusing attention on threat in any given situation and overestimating risk (Peters et al., 2014), and with a range of cognitive and reasoning biases (Garety and Freeman, 2013).

Recent developments in CBTp for delusions include a move towards focusing on putative causal or maintenance factors of delusions, such as rumination and worry, insomnia, negative self-beliefs, reasoning biases, and safety behaviours, in a bid to understand the most effective mechanisms of change in CBT for delusions (Freeman, 2016; Garety et al., 2015). This approach is outlined in the section on 'Does cognitive behaviour therapy for psychosis work? Efficacy and effectiveness' in more detail when the evidence for CBTp is discussed.

Cognitive behaviour therapy for hallucinations

Hallucinations in psychosis are most commonly auditory verbal in form; consequently, the majority of evaluations report on interventions for voice-hearing. Similar to the aims of intervention with delusions, the goal is not necessarily to get rid of voices, nor to challenge their reality. Sometimes it may be possible to alter the negative content of voices (for example, if they reflect negative automatic thoughts or depressed mood), but for many neither their frequency nor their content can be changed. Instead, the central tenets of therapy are: (1) to modify the beliefs the person holds about their voices relating to their perceived omnipotence and malevolence (Chadwick and Birchwood, 1994), to reduce distress and unhelpful behaviours (such as complying with command hallucinations (Birchwood et al., 2014) and improve functioning, according to jointly agreed goals; and (2) to change their relationship with their voices to enhance their self-esteem and reduce the power imbalance (Birchwood et al., 2000). Again, all therapeutic work is based on the formulation, including making links with the client's personal history, especially past experiences of psychological trauma, bullying, and victimization, which are often reflected in voice content, directly or thematically. Triggers and maintenance factors, for both the experiences and their appraisals, are identified and targeted, and coping strategies are enhanced to increase perceived control. Safety behaviours are gently discouraged, with the aim of weakening the perceived omniscience and omnipotence of voices. Non-adversarial testing of the voice's predictions, knowledge, and threats is encouraged. An important aspect of the therapeutic work consists of bolstering the person's self-esteem and reducing 'social-rank threat', i.e. unhelpful schemas about the self and others and one's position in the social world as subordinate and inferior (Birchwood et al., 2004; Meaden et al., 2012).

Recent developments in CBT for voices include: targeting the distress associated with auditory hallucinations by increasing the person's assertiveness with their voices, family, and social environment (Hayward et al., 2017); conducting therapy with avatars, where distressing voices are digitally represented so voice-hearers can be visually 'exposed' to and have a controlled dialogue with their persecuting voices, with the aim of reducing their impact (Craig et al., 2018); and focusing on the reduction of harmful compliance with voices through changing the voice power differential (Birchwood et al., 2014; 2017). There have also been developments in cognitive models linking voices to traumatic past experiences, which have clear clinical applications (Hardy, 2017; Berry et al., 2017).

Delivery of cognitive behaviour therapy for psychosis

In the UK, NICE guidance (National Institute of Health and Care Excellence, 2017) recommends that CBTp should be offered to all people with psychosis. The guidance is based on the results of clinical trials of CBTp and recommends adherence to cognitive models, through the use of detailed protocols in routine clinical practice, to increase the likelihood that the outcomes will match, as closely as possible, the outcomes achieved in clinical trials.

Adherence to CBTp models can be evaluated through the process of monitoring therapy content and rating session recordings for fidelity to CBTp models on a general cognitive therapy rating scale and scales measuring specific CBTp items (Rollinson et al., 2008; Startup et al., 2002; Fowler et al., 2011; Blackburn et al., 2001). Necessary therapist competencies to deliver CBTp, which are based on the current available evidence for the effectiveness of approaches and interventions, have been outlined (Roth and Pilling, 2013).

In practice there is variation in the number and frequency of sessions attended, and the rate at which the therapy elements are addressed, such as time to agreeing a therapy goal, sharing individualized formulations, and interventions such as cognitive or behavioural change strategies (Morrison, 2017). However, NICE guidance recommends a minimum of 16 sessions of CBTp over a 6–9-month period for adults experiencing distressing psychotic symptoms (National Institute of Health and Care Excellence, 2017).

What outcomes do service-users value?

Brabban and colleagues (Brabban et al., 2016) reported the results of three separate syntheses of qualitative research into the experience of receiving CBTp (Berry and Hayward, 2011; Holding et al., 2016; Wood et al., 2015), all of which reported on service-user valued aspects of CBTp. In summary, improvement in symptoms, including distressing beliefs, voices, mood, anxiety, and self-esteem, were valued, along with developing acceptance of, and an ability to cope with, psychotic experiences. Improvements in social and occupational functioning and the development of hope were also identified as important positive outcomes of CBTp. The collaborative development of an individual case formulation between therapist and client was consistently endorsed as an important process for facilitating a change in understanding psychotic experiences and to view them in the context of the individual's life experiences. The importance of a good therapeutic relationship in which these changes could occur was considered crucial (Holding et al., 2016; Wood et al., 2015).

Does cognitive behaviour therapy for psychosis work? Efficacy and effectiveness

The majority of randomized controlled trials (RCTs) have evaluated composite CBTp approaches for mixed groups of patients. Therapy could address psychotic experiences, affective disturbance, problematic schemas, social functioning, or relapse prevention, depending on presenting difficulties, often necessitating measurement of multiple outcomes. Therapy could be provided in a range of formats, such as group or individual, and last anything between a few sessions to over a year. There have been more than 20 meta-analyses reviewing up to 50 RCTs, with effect sizes across the different meta-analyses ranging from small to large, but, overall, averaging around 0.40. Results are less consistent for the smaller number of studies comparing CBTp with other psychological interventions (Van Der Gaag et al., 2014; Mehl et al., 2015; Kennedy and Xyrichis, 2017), and there is a need to strengthen the evidence base for CBTp compared to an alternative therapy with adequately powered trials (Jones et al., 2004; Lynch et al., 2010). Although less rigorous than RCTs, there is also a developing 'practice-based evidence', with studies of CBTp delivered in routine settings demonstrating overall effectiveness (Krakvik et al., 2013; Lincoln et al., 2012; Morrison et al., 2004; Peters et al., 2010), and that the therapeutic effects for specific psychotic symptoms found in RCTs are not diluted by delivery in routine services (Morrison et al., 2004; Peters et al., 2015; Jolley et al., 2015). However, two of the larger meta-analyses reported an inverse relationship between effect size and methodological rigour, especially blinding (Jauhar et al., 2014; Wykes et al., 2008), suggesting caution in interpreting positive outcomes of CBTp.

Nevertheless, it can be problematic to interpret the effect sizes presented in meta-analyses owing to the heterogeneity of presenting problems, whether therapy was provided in individual or group format, and because of a range of different intervention targets (Byrne, 2014; Peters, 2014). While this approach can address whether there is an overall effect, it does not permit answers to specific questions of what works for whom or show where improvements in treatments are required (Thomas, 2015). Establishing an evidence base for CBTp has relied on the adoption of drug trial methodology to establish credibility, overcome resistance to offering therapy to this group, and show that CBTp is safe, acceptable, and effective (Brabban et al., 2016). While this approach has been crucial in leading to the inclusion of CBTp in international healthcare guidance recommendations, thereby enabling its translation into routine clinical practice, it has not been free of criticism. For instance, Birchwood and others have suggested that it is not appropriate to evaluate CBTp as if it were a 'quasi-neuroleptic' (Byrne, 2014; Birchwood and Trower, 2006; Thomas, 2015), when the main focus of CBTp is on the emotional and behavioural impact of psychotic symptoms and not on their frequency or severity (Birchwood, 2003). The use of a broad assessment tool such as the Positive And Negative Symptom Scale (PANSS) (Kay et al., 1987), the 'gold standard' outcome measure for antipsychotic trial protocols, covers more symptom areas than are targeted in therapy, while at the same time failing to capture the nuanced dimensional changes expected in CBTp, such as preoccupation about delusions or power beliefs about voices. It therefore lacks sensitivity to individual outcomes while providing trials with 'an insensitive test of the null hypothesis that CBTp does nothing at all' (Thomas, 2015). In practice, CBTp targets different areas depending on the individual's goals and formulation, which may lead to a dilution of effects as people improve in different domains. Studies where the research strategy was to target specific symptoms, mechanisms, or components of CBTp, and evaluate the outcomes being targeted, such as voice distress or associated behaviour, have shown higher effect sizes (Lincoln and Peters, 2018). These studies reflect a recent move towards targeted interventions, focusing on specific symptoms or putative causal or maintenance factors, examining and targeting discrete components according to the interventionist causal model approach (Kendler and Campbell, 2009) outlined by Freeman (Freeman, 2011; Freeman et al., 2016b). Freeman and colleagues have used this approach with persecutory delusions and have found that interventions to reduce worry and rumination (Freeman et al., 2015a) and virtual reality cognitive therapy to address safety behaviours (Freeman et al., 2016a) can be effective in reducing delusional conviction. Further pilot investigation of CBT for insomnia (Freeman et al., 2015b) and negative self-cognitions in people with persecutory delusions did not identify a significant impact on delusional conviction, although larger trials are warranted. Studies have shown that improving reasoning skills and increasing belief flexibility (Garety et al., 2015; Waller et al., 2015) also improves persecutory delusions. Freeman and colleagues are conducting a trial of a modular treatment for persecutory delusions (the 'Feeling Safe Programme'), where service-users choose from a range of CBT protocols to target each of the putative causal or maintenance factors of delusions (Freeman et al., 2016c).

Cognitive behaviour therapy for psychosis outcomes for people who do not respond to medication

The most robust evidence base for CBTp is for people who are medication treatment-resistant. Burns and colleagues (Burns et al., 2014) conducted a meta-analysis examining the effectiveness of CBTp among outpatients with medication-resistant psychosis, both on completion of therapy and at follow-up. The estimated effect size for reduction in positive symptoms (summarizing the findings of 16 studies) was 0.47 at the end of therapy and 0.41 at follow-up. The authors noted that the results were limited to trials including well-trained and experienced psychologists with expertise in CBTp. A larger multicentre RCT, including 487 participants (Pyle et al., 2016), is currently under way to investigate further the limited evidence for CBTp's effectiveness for those 'for whom an adequate trial of clozapine has either not been possible due to tolerability problems or was not associated with a sufficient therapeutic response' (Pyle et al., 2016).

Cognitive behaviour therapy for psychosis outcomes for those who choose not to take medication

A number of people choose not to take or discontinue antipsychotic medication for a range of reasons (Wade et al., 2017). Morrison and colleagues (Morrison et al., 2014) conducted a pilot, single-blind RCT of 74 individuals with schizophrenia spectrum disorders who had chosen not to take medication to examine whether CBTp was efficacious in this group. The results were promising. There was evidence for a reduction of symptoms in the CBTp group, and therapy was considered safe and acceptable. Criticism of the study included that the participants had less severe symptoms than those usually participating in acute drug trials, and the study did not include an active therapy control group (Howes, 2014). The first pilot trial to compare CBTp directly to antipsychotic medication and to a combination of both CBTp and antipsychotic medication (Law et al., 2017) is under way. The outcome of this trial will provide a better understanding of the range of treatment advice that should be offered to people with psychosis who are unwilling or unable to take antipsychotic medication.

Factors influencing cognitive behaviour therapy for psychosis outcomes

Approximately half of those offered CBTp show improvements in psychotic symptoms (Wykes et al., 2008). There is limited evidence regarding the specific CBTp techniques contributing to positive changes during therapy; however, therapeutic alliance has consistently been shown to be important (Goldsmith et al., 2015; Jung et al., 2014). High-quality training and delivery of CBTp specific interventions are necessary to achieve positive outcomes (Steel et al., 2012; Jolley et al., 2015). While NICE guidelines suggest a minimum of 16 sessions, researchers (Lincoln et al., 2016) have identified that significant symptom improvement and reduction in distress takes place by session 15, while the frequency of positive and negative symptoms reach a minimum by session 25. Data from large clinical trials (Flach et al., 2015; Dunn et al., 2012) suggest that components of CBTp, such as collaboratively agreed goals for therapy, individualized problem formulation, active change strategies, and between-session tasks, contribute to better outcomes. In addition, illness perceptions were associated with therapy engagement, in that patients who took up full therapy were more likely to attribute the cause of their problems to their personality and state of mind (Freeman et al., 2013) rather than to biological causes. A lack of insight and poor social functioning were associated with drop-out in CBTp (Lincoln et al., 2014), while better coping skills (Premkumar et al., 2011) were associated with better outcomes. A recent systematic review examining which factors predict favourable outcome in CBTp (O'Keeffe et al., 2017) identified female gender, older age, higher clinical insight at baseline, shorter duration of the illness, and higher educational attainment as predictive of favourable outcome in CBTp.

Conclusions

There is a consistent evidence base to indicate that CBTp is an effective adjunctive therapy to medication for those with persisting positive symptoms of psychosis. There is also tentative evidence to suggest that people who choose not to take antipsychotic medication can benefit from CBTp (Morrison et al., 2014), and whether it can be considered as an alternative treatment to medication is currently being investigated (Law et al., 2017). The outcomes of this research will be important to facilitate informed treatment choices in this service-user group (Howes, 2014). CBTp is broadly seen as an acceptable, helpful, and positive experience by service-users (Brabban et al., 2016). Recent developments in CBTp include targeting putative causal and maintenance factors of persecutory delusions (Freeman, 2016; Garety et al., 2015) and developments in approaches to, and understanding of, voices (Berry et al., 2017; Hayward et al., 2017; Birchwood et al., 2014; Craig et al., 2018) and trauma (Hardy, 2017). CBTp research continues to highlight the processes involved in the development and maintenance of positive psychotic symptoms, how these can best be addressed in therapy, and what works best for whom.

REFERENCES

Bentall, R. P., Fernyhough, C., Morrison, A. P., Lewis, S., Corcoran, R. (2007). Prospects for a cognitive-developmental account of psychotic experiences. *Br J Clin Psychol, 46,* 155–73.

Berry, C., Hayward, M. (2011). What can qualitative research tell us about service user perspectives of CBT for psychosis? A synthesis of current evidence. *Behav Cogn Psychother, 39,* 487–94.

Berry, K., Varese, F., Bucci, S. (2017). Cognitive attachment model of voices: evidence base and future implications. *Front Psychiatry, 8,* 111.

Birchwood, M., Meaden, A., Trower, P., Gilbert, P., Plaistow, J. (2000). The power and omnipotence of voices: subordination and entrapment by voices and significant others. *Psychol Med, 30,* 337–44.

Birchwood, M. (2003). Pathways to emotional dysfunction in first-episode psychosis. *Br J Psychiatry*, 182, 373–5.

Birchwood, M., Trower, P. (2006). The future of cognitive-behavioural therapy for psychosis: not a quasi-neuroleptic. *Br J Psychiatry*, 188, 107–8.

Birchwood, M., Gilbert, P., Gilbert, J., et al. (2004). Interpersonal and role-related schema influence the relationship with the dominant 'voice' in schizophrenia: a comparison of three models. *Psychol Med*, 34, 1571–80.

Birchwood, M., Michail, M., Meaden, A., et al. (2014). Cognitive behaviour therapy to prevent harmful compliance with command hallucinations (COMMAND): a randomised controlled trial. *Lancet Psychiatry*, 1, 23–33.

Birchwood, M., Dunn, G., Meaden, A., et al. (2017). The COMMAND trial of cognitive therapy to prevent harmful compliance with command hallucinations: predictors of outcome and mediators of change. *Psychol Med*, Dec 5, 1–9. doi: 10.1017/S0033291717003488. [Epub ahead of print]

Blackburn, I. M., James, I. A., Milne, D. L., et al. (2001). The Revised Cognitive Therapy Scale (CTS-R): psychometric properties. *Behav Cogn Psychother*, 29, 431–46.

Brabban, A., Byrne, R., Longden, E., Morrison, A. P. (2016). The importance of human relationships, ethics and recovery-orientated values in the delivery of CBT for people with psychosis. *Psychosis*, 9, 157–66.

Burns, A. M., Erickson, D. H., Brenner, C. A. (2014). Cognitive-behavioral therapy for medication-resistant psychosis: a meta-analytic review. *Psychiatr Serv*, 65, 874–80.

Byrne, R. E. (2014). CBT for psychosis: not a 'quasi-neuroleptic'. *Br J Psychiatry*, 204, 489.

Chadwick, P., Birchwood, M. (1994). The omnipotence of voices. A cognitive approach to auditory hallucinations. *Br J Psychiatry*, 164, 190–201.

Chadwick, P., Birchwood, M., Tower, P. (1996). *Cognitive Therapy for Delusions, Voices and Paranoia*. Chichester: Wiley.

Craig, T. K., Rus-Calafell, M., Ward, T., et al. (2018). AVATAR therapy for auditory verbal hallucinations in people with psychosis: a single-blind, randomised controlled trial. *Lancet Psychiatry*, 5, 31–40.

Dunn, G., Fowler, D., Rollinson, R., et al. (2012). Effective elements of cognitive behaviour therapy for psychosis: results of a novel type of subgroup analysis based on principal stratification. *Psychol Med*, 42, 1057–68.

Flach, C., French, P., Dunn, G., et al. (2015). Components of therapy as mechanisms of change in cognitive therapy for people at risk of psychosis: analysis of the EDIE-2 trial. *Br J Psychiatry*, 207, 123–9.

Fowler, D., Garety, P., Kuipers, E. (1995). *Cognitive Behaviour Therapy for Psychosis: theory and practice*. Chichester: Wiley.

Fowler, D., Rollinson, R., French, P. (2011). Adherence and competence assessment in studies of CBT for psychosis: current status and future directions. *Epidemiol Psychiatr Sci*, 20, 121–6.

Freeman, D. (2011). Improving cognitive treatments for delusions. *Schizophr Res*, 132, 135–9.

Freeman, D. (2016). Persecutory delusions: a cognitive perspective on understanding and treatment. *Lancet Psychiatry,* 3, 685–92.

Freeman, D., Garety, P. A. (2003). Connecting neurosis and psychosis: the direct influence of emotion on delusions and hallucinations. *Behav Res Ther,* 41, 923–47.

Freeman, D., Garety, P. A., Kuipers, E., Fowler, D., Bebbington, P. E. (2002). A cognitive model of persecutory delusions. *Br J Clin Psychol,* 41, 331–47.

Freeman, D., Freeman, J., Garety, P. A. (2006). *Overcoming Paranoid and Suspicious Thoughts.* London: Constable and Robinson.

Freeman, D., Bentall, R., Garety, P. (2008). *Persecutory Delusions: assessment, theory, and treatment.* Oxford: Oxford University Press.

Freeman, D., Dunn, G., Garety, P., et al. (2013). Patients' beliefs about the causes, persistence and control of psychotic experiences predict take-up of effective cognitive behaviour therapy for psychosis. *Psychol Med,* 43, 269–77.

Freeman, D., Dunn, G., Startup, H., et al. (2015a). Effects of cognitive behaviour therapy for worry on persecutory delusions in patients with psychosis (WIT): a parallel, single-blind, randomised controlled trial with a mediation analysis. *Lancet Psychiatry,* 2, 305–13.

Freeman, D., Waite, F., Startup, H., et al. (2015b). Efficacy of cognitive behavioural therapy for sleep improvement in patients with persistent delusions and hallucinations (BEST): a prospective, assessor-blind, randomised controlled pilot trial. *Lancet Psychiatry,* 2, 975–83.

Freeman, D., Bradley, J., Antley, A., et al. (2016a). Virtual reality in the treatment of persecutory delusions: randomised controlled experimental study testing how to reduce delusional conviction. *Br J Psychiatry,* 209, 62–7.

Freeman, D., Bradley, J., Waite, F., et al. (2016b). Targeting recovery in persistent persecutory delusions: a proof of principle study of a new translational psychological treatment (the Feeling Safe Programme). *Behav Cogn Psychother,* 44, 539–52.

Freeman, D., Waite, F., Emsley, R., et al. (2016c). The efficacy of a new translational treatment for persecutory delusions: study protocol for a randomised controlled trial (The Feeling Safe Study). *Trials,* 17, 134.

French, P., Morrison, A. P. (2004). *Early Detection and Cognitive Therapy for People at High Risk of Developing Psychosis: a treatment approach.* Chichester: John Wiley & Sons.

Garety, P., Waller, H., Emsley, R., et al. (2015). Cognitive mechanisms of change in delusions: an experimental investigation targeting reasoning to effect change in paranoia. *Schizophr Bull,* 41, 400–10.

Garety, P. A., Freeman, D. (2013). The past and future of delusions research: from the inexplicable to the treatable. *Br J Psychiatry,* 203, 327–33.

Garety, P. A., Kuipers, E., Fowler, D., Freeman, D., Bebbington, P. E. (2001). A cognitive model of the positive symptoms of psychosis. *Psychol Med,* 31, 189–95.

Garety, P. A., Bebbington, P., Fowler, D., Freeman, D., Kuipers, E. (2007). Implications for neurobiological research of cognitive models of psychosis: a theoretical paper. *Psychol Med,* 37, 1377–91.

Goldsmith, L. P., Lewis, S. W., Dunn, G., Bentall, R. P. (2015). Psychological treatments for early psychosis can be beneficial or harmful, depending on the therapeutic alliance: an instrumental variable analysis. *Psychol Med,* 45, 2365–73.

Gumley, A., Schwannauer, M. (2006). *Staying Well After Psychosis.* Chichester: John Wiley & Sons.

Hardy, A. (2017). Pathways from trauma to psychotic experiences: a theoretically informed model of posttraumatic stress in psychosis. *Front Psychol,* 8, 697.

Hayward, M., Strauss, D., Kingdon, D. (2012). *Overcoming Distressing Voices.* London: Constable and Robinson.

Hayward, M., Jones, A. M., Bogen-Johnston, L., Thomas, N., Strauss, C. (2017). Relating therapy for distressing auditory hallucinations: a pilot randomized controlled trial. *Schizophr Res,* 183, 137–42.

Holding, J. C., Gregg, L., Haddock, G. (2016). Individuals' experiences and opinions of psychological therapies for psychosis: a narrative synthesis. *Clin Psychol Rev,* 43, 142–61.

Howes, O. (2014). Cognitive therapy: at last an alternative to antipsychotics? *Lancet,* 383, 1364–6.

Hunter, E., Johns, L., Onwumere, J., Peters, E. (2014). Cognitive behavioural therapy for psychosis. In: Buckley, P. F., Gaughran, F. (eds) *Treatment-Refractory Schizophrenia.* Berlin-Heidelberg: Springer-Verlag.

Jauhar, S., Mckenna, P. J., Radua, J., Fung, E., Salvador, R., Laws, K. R. (2014). Cognitive-behavioural therapy for the symptoms of schizophrenia: systematic review and meta-analysis with examination of potential bias. *Br J Psychiatry,* 204, 20–9.

Jolley, S., Garety, P., Peters, E., et al. (2015). Opportunities and challenges in Improving Access to Psychological Therapies for people with Severe Mental Illness (IAPT-SMI): evaluating the first operational year of the South London and Maudsley (SLaM) demonstration site for psychosis. *Behav Res Ther,* 64, 24–30.

Jones, C., Cormac, I., Silveira Da Mota Neto, J. I., Campbell, C. (2004). Cognitive behaviour therapy for schizophrenia. *Cochrane Database Syst Rev,* CD000524.

Jung, E., Wiesjahn, M., Lincoln, T. M. (2014). Negative, not positive symptoms predict the early therapeutic alliance in cognitive behavioral therapy for psychosis. *Psychother Res,* 24, 171–83.

Kay, S. R., Fiszbein, A., Opler, L. A. (1987). The Positive And Negative Syndrome Scale (PANSS) for schizophrenia. *Schizophr Bull,* 13, 261–76.

Kendler, K. S., Campbell, J. (2009). Interventionist causal models in psychiatry: repositioning the mind-body problem. *Psychol Med,* 39, 881–7.

Kennedy, L., Xyrichis, A. (2017). Cognitive behavioral therapy compared with non-specialized therapy for alleviating the effect of auditory hallucinations in people with reoccurring schizophrenia: a systematic review and meta-analysis. *Community Ment Health J,* 53, 127–33.

Kingdon, D., Turkington, D. (1994). *Cognitive Behaviour Therapy of Schizophrenia.* New York: Guilford Press.

Krakvik, B., Grawe, R. W., Hagen, R., Stiles, T. C. (2013). Cognitive behaviour therapy for psychotic symptoms: a randomized controlled effectiveness trial. *Behav Cogn Psychother,* 41, 511–24.

CHAPTER 11

Law, H., Carter, L., Sellers, R., et al. (2017). A pilot randomised controlled trial comparing antipsychotic medication to cognitive behavioural therapy to a combination of both in people with psychosis: rationale, study design and baseline data of the COMPARE trial. *Psychosis*, 9, 193–204.

Lincoln, T. M., Peters, E. (2018). A systematic review and discussion of symptom specific cognitive behavioural approaches to delusions and hallucinations. *Schizophr Res*, Jan 16. pii: S0920-9964(17)30766-1. doi: 10.1016/j.schres.2017.12.014. [Epub ahead of print].

Lincoln, T. M., Ziegler, M., Mehl, S., et al. (2012). Moving from efficacy to effectiveness in cognitive behavioral therapy for psychosis: a randomized clinical practice trial. *J Consult Clin Psychol*, 80, 674–86.

Lincoln, T. M., Rief, W., Westermann, S., et al. (2014). Who stays, who benefits? Predicting dropout and change in cognitive behaviour therapy for psychosis. *Psychiatry Res*, 216, 198–205.

Lincoln, T. M., Jung, E., Wiesjahn, M., Schlier, B. (2016). What is the minimal dose of cognitive behavior therapy for psychosis? An approximation using repeated assessments over 45 sessions. *Eur Psychiatry*, 38, 31–9.

Lynch, D., Laws, K. R., Mckenna, P. J. (2010). Cognitive behavioural therapy for major psychiatric disorder: does it really work? A meta-analytical review of well-controlled trials. *Psychol Med*, 40, 9–24.

Meaden, A., Keen, N., Aston, R., Barton, K., Bucci, S. (2012). *Cognitive Therapy for Command Hallucinations: an advanced practical companion*. Hove: Routledge.

Mehl, S., Werner, D., Lincoln, T. M. (2015). Does Cognitive Behavior Therapy for psychosis (CBTp) show a sustainable effect on delusions? A meta-analysis. *Front Psychol*, 6, 1450.

Morris, E., Johns, L., Oliver, J. (2013). *Acceptance and Commitment Therapy and Mindfullness for Psychosis*. Chichester: Wiley-Blackwell.

Morrison, A. P. (2001). The interpretation of intrusions in psychosis: an integrative cognitive approach to psychotic symptoms. *Beh CognPsychother*, 29, 257–76.

Morrison, A. P. (2017). A manualised treatment protocol to guide delivery of evidence-based cognitive therapy for people with distressing psychosis: learning from clinical trials. *Psychosis*, 9, 271–81.

Morrison, A. P., Barratt, S. (2010). What are the components of CBT for psychosis? A Delphi study. *Schizophr Bull*, 36, 136–42.

Morrison, A. P., Renton, J. C., Williams, S., et al. (2004). Delivering cognitive therapy to people with psychosis in a community mental health setting: an effectiveness study. *Acta Psychiatr Scand*, 110, 36–44.

Morrison, A. P., Turkington, D., Pyle, M., et al. (2014). Cognitive therapy for people with schizophrenia spectrum disorders not taking antipsychotic drugs: a single-blind randomised controlled trial. *Lancet*, 383, 1395–403.

National Institute of Health and Care Excellence. (2017). Surveillance report 2017- *Psychosis and Schizophrenia in Adults: prevention and management* (2014) NICE Guideline CG178. London: NICE.

O'Keeffe, J., Conway, R., McGuire, B. (2017). A systematic review examining factors predicting favourable outcome in cognitive behavioural interventions for psychosis. *Schizophr Res*, 183, 22–30.

Peters, E. (2014). An oversimplification of psychosis, its treatment, and its outcomes? *Br J Psychiatry*, 205, 159–60.

Peters, E., Landau, S., McCrone, P., et al. (2010). A randomised controlled trial of cognitive behaviour therapy for psychosis in a routine clinical service. *Acta Psychiatr Scand*, 122, 302–18.

Peters, E., Crombie, T., Agbedjro, D., et al. (2015). The long-term effectiveness of cognitive behavior therapy for psychosis within a routine psychological therapies service. *Front Psychol*, 6, 1658.

Peters, E. R., Moritz, S., Schwannauer, M., et al. (2014). Cognitive biases questionnaire for psychosis. *Schizophr Bull*, 40, 300–13.

Premkumar, P., Peters, E. R., Fannon, D., Anilkumar, A. P., Kuipers, E., Kumari, V. (2011). Coping styles predict responsiveness to cognitive behaviour therapy in psychosis. *Psychiatry Res*, 187, 354–62.

Pyle, M., Norrie, J., Schwannauer, M. (2016). Design and protocol for the Focusing on Clozapine Unresponsive Symptoms (FOCUS) trial: a randomised controlled trial. *BMC Psychiatry*, 16, 280.

Rollinson, R., Smith, B., Steel, C., et al. (2008). Measuring adherence in CBT for psychosis: a psychometric analysis of an adherence scale. *Behav Cogn Psychother*, 36, 163–78.

Roth, A., Pilling, S. (2013). *A Competence Framework for Psychological Interventions with People with Psychosis and Bipolar Disorder*. London: University College London.

Startup, M., Jackson, M., Pearce, E. (2002). Assessing therapist adherence to cognitive-behaviour therapy for psychosis. *Behav Cogn Psychother*, 30, 329–39.

Steel, C., Tarrier, N., Stahl, D., Wykes, T. (2012). Cognitive behaviour therapy for psychosis: the impact of therapist training and supervision. *Psychother Psychosom*, 81, 194–5.

Thomas, N. (2015). What's really wrong with cognitive behavioral therapy for psychosis? *Front Psychol*, 6, 323.

Van Der Gaag, M., Van Den Berg, D., Nieman, D. (2013). *CBT for Those at Risk of a First Episode Psychosis*. Hove: Routledge.

Van Der Gaag, M., Valmaggia, L. R., Smit, F. (2014). The effects of individually tailored formulation-based cognitive behavioural therapy in auditory hallucinations and delusions: a meta-analysis. *Schizophr Res*, 156, 30–7.

Wade, M., Tai, S., Awenat, Y., Haddock, G. (2017). A systematic review of service-user reasons for adherence and nonadherence to neuroleptic medication in psychosis. *Clin Psychol Rev*, 51, 75–95.

Waller, H., Emsley, R., Freeman, D., et al. (2015). Thinking well: a randomised controlled feasibility study of a new CBT therapy targeting reasoning biases in people with distressing persecutory delusional beliefs. *J Behav Ther Exp Psychiatry*, 48, 82–9.

Wood, L., Burke, E., Morrison, A. (2015). Individual cognitive behavioural therapy for psychosis (CBTp): a systematic review of qualitative literature. *Behav Cogn Psychother*, 43, 285–97.

CHAPTER 11

Wright, N. P., Turkington, D., Kelly, O. P., et al. (2014). *A Clinician's Guide to Integrating Acceptance and Commitment Therapy, Compassion-Focused Therapy, and Mindfulness Approaches within the Cognitive Behavioral Therapy Tradition.* Oakland, CA: New Harbinger.

Wykes, T., Steel, C., Everitt, B., Tarrier, N. (2008). Cognitive behavior therapy for schizophrenia: effect sizes, clinical models, and methodological rigor. *Schizophr Bull,* 34, 523–37.

CHAPTER 12

Ultra-treatment resistance

Gary Remington, Ofer Agid, Hiroyoshi Takeuchi, Jimmy Lee, and Araba Chintoh

---

KEY POINTS

- In schizophrenia, the term ultra-treatment resistance is generally used to refer to an illness that has shown an inadequate response to an adequate trial of clozapine in the absence of other confounding factors that might compromise response (e.g. substance abuse, antipsychotic non-adherence). It is more precisely termed clozapine (ultra-medication) resistance or clozapine-resistant schizophrenia (CRS).

- A number of drug treatment strategies have been evaluated for ultra-treatment resistance, including adding a second antipsychotic to clozapine, mood stabilizers, and glutamate modulators.

- Whilst there is trial evidence to support a number of these strategies, robust, meta-analytic data are generally lacking. Where they are tried, it is important to evaluate response carefully and discontinue a treatment if there is not clear evidence for a benefit that outweighs side effects.

- There is evidence of a robust benefit of electroconvulsive therapy in patients with ultra-treatment resistance taking clozapine, although many of the studies were open label.

- Ultra-treatment resistance is heterogeneous, and so it is unlikely that one treatment will be effective for all patients.

The central role of clozapine in ultra-resistant schizophrenia

Clozapine has established itself as the only antipsychotic with proven efficacy in treatment-resistant schizophrenia (TRS), a point captured within current treatment algorithms and guidelines (Warnez and Alessi-Severini, 2014). This said, clozapine is not a panacea for TRS; response in the early controlled trials ranged from 30% to 60%, with a more recent meta-analysis reporting a figure of 40% (Siskind et al., 2017). As a result, we have witnessed a growing literature on alternatives to clozapine (or lack thereof), as well as augmentation strategies in the case of suboptimal clozapine response (Dold and Leucht, 2014; Englisch and Zink, 2012; Kristensen et al., 2013; Miyamoto et al., 2014; Samara et al., 2016).

Clozapine-resistant or ultra-resistant schizophrenia

Criteria

The term 'ultra-resistant schizophrenia' (URS) gained a foothold when, in a review of clozapine augmentation in 2006, criteria were detailed that defined individuals who were clozapine-refractory and were therefore candidates for other treatments (Mouaffak et al., 2006). These are outlined in Table 12.1, as are the criteria of one additional report since that addresses this same topic (Lee et al., 2015b).

The criteria for URS follow similar principles to those established for TRS. For example, they too address clinical eligibility, what constitutes an adequate trial, and threshold for efficacy (Brenner et al., 1990; Conley and Buchanan, 1997; Itil et al., 1966; Kane et al., 1988; Suzuki et al., 2012). However, there are differences. Antipsychotic dosing thresholds are detailed for TRS and, in fact, have been reduced over the years (Conley and Buchanan, 1997) in the face of evidence: a) challenging the value of high antipsychotic doses (Baldessarini et al., 1988; Bollini et al., 1994; Davis and Chen, 2004); and b) the identification of D_2-related thresholds through

Table 12.1 Comparison of published criteria for ultra-resistant or clozapine-resistant schizophrenia

Criteria	Mouaffak et al., 2006	Lee et al., 2015b
Adequate dose	Plasma levels >350 ng/mL	Plasma level ≥350 ng/mL for once a day dosing[a]; ≥250 ng/mL for equal divided dosing or oral doses ≥400 mg/day
Adequate duration (weeks)	8	8, at adequate dose
No significant improvement	<20% decrease on BPRS	CGI-SCH positive change >2 (2 = much improved)
Current illness severity	BPRS ≥45, CGI-S ≥4, and ≥4 on at least two out of four positive items on the BPRS	CGI-SCH positive ≥4 (4 = moderately ill)
Duration of illness with no good functioning (years)	5	Not applicable

[a]Plasma levels should be taken after 5 days of unchanged clozapine dosing and 12 hours from last clozapine dose.

BPRS, Brief Psychiatric Rating Scale; CGI–S, Clinical Global Impression-Severity; CGI–SCH, Clinical Global Impression-Schizophrenia.

neuroimaging, evidence that could be used to establish optimal clinical dosing and, in addition, allow for comparison between agents (Kapur et al., 2000). Clozapine's pharmacology is not conducive to this strategy (Kapur et al., 1999), and even now what constitutes clinically appropriate doses remains unclear (Subramanian et al., 2017). Accordingly, both sets of available criteria have embraced plasma levels (i.e. therapeutic drug monitoring) as an option to specific doses, although the evidence in this regard is 'soft', compromised by considerable interindividual as well as intraindividual variability (Guitton et al., 1999; Lee et al., 2016).

Several other differences warrant comment, and these distinguish the two sets of URS criteria that have been published. While the original URS criteria incorporated a global measure of improvement for confirmation of treatment response (i.e. 20% decrease), the more recent criteria have suggested that treatment response be confined to improvement in positive symptoms. The basis for this argument is twofold. In clinical reality, it is persistent psychosis that shapes clinicians' impressions of illness severity and response to treatment (Lee et al., 2015a). Moreover, evidence that clozapine is particularly unique in terms of other major symptom domains associated with schizophrenia (e.g. cognitive, negative) has not been forthcoming (Lee et al., 2015a; Nielsen et al., 2015). The position taken by the newer criteria is that the focus be positive symptoms, the symptom domain central to TRS as well as URS (Lee et al., 2015a; 2015b). In doing so, this also maintains clarity from the standpoint of new treatment development, whether it be drug or otherwise. We are reminded of the broad claims that were made regarding improvement with the advent of second-generation antipsychotics, claims that were not substantiated as evidence accrued (Remington, 2003). The notion of a 'silver bullet' treatment for schizophrenia's multiple symptom domains belies the illness's complexity (Remington et al., 2012). This does not negate the position that other symptom domains may also be treatment-resistant; indeed, current evidence would suggest this, at least with regard to cognitive and negative symptoms (Fusar-Poli et al., 2015; Hagan and Jones, 2005; Marder, 2006; Remington et al., 2012). The field will be better served, however, if the domains are kept separate, although this then calls for changes in terminology specific to the use of treatment resistance. Again, though, this may also prove useful as we move toward personalized medicine and the recognition that individuals will each bring unique combinations of symptoms that need to be treated differently. Terminology will be discussed further in the section on 'Terminology'.

Returning to existing URS criteria, the more recent report also omits the use of a criterion that brings into play functioning and duration of illness. The original URS criteria, as well as criteria for the seminal clozapine work in TRS, both included a criterion that requires illness duration of at least 5 years in association with poor functioning (Kane et al., 1988; Mouaffak et al., 2006). However, current evidence suggesting that early and effective treatment in schizophrenia is associated with improved treatment outcome (Rubio and Correll, 2017) would argue strongly against a 5-year delay in access to clozapine. In fact, existing evidence specific to clozapine, TRS, and delayed treatment seems to support this position (Ucok et al., 2015; Yada et al., 2015; Yoshimura et al., 2017). Notably, though, while clozapine is effective in the treatment of schizophrenia's positive symptoms, this does not necessarily translate to occupational and social functioning (Lee et al., 2014).

Terminology

TRS as a descriptor has been challenged as fostering therapeutic nihilism, and the term 'neuroleptic-resistant schizophrenia' forwarded as a more optimistic option (Williams et al., 2002). Taking this a step further, there is an argument that both these terms are incorrect since at least a portion of this population will respond to clozapine, raising the alternative that TRS is better termed 'clozapine-eligible schizophrenia' (CES) (Lee et al., 2015b). This is certainly less nihilistic and takes into account the fact that a number of individuals may not receive clozapine although they fall within a group that meets criteria for such a trial. It also represents important information for clinicians in their decisions regarding treatment and assumptions regarding response. Those who have an adequate trial of clozapine, but demonstrate a suboptimal response, are the only individuals who represent URS, a descriptor that is technically correct but arguably even more nihilistic than TRS, as for these individuals there is no treatment with clear evidence of clinical superiority (see section on 'Treatment'). Aligning with the descriptor CES, it has been proposed that clozapine-resistant schizophrenia (CRS) may represent a more accurate descriptor than URS, confirming that an adequate trial with clozapine has been undertaken and proven suboptimal in terms of response (Lee et al., 2015b).

Fig. 12.1 details the antipsychotic treatment of schizophrenia, including clozapine's position in treatment trials, as well as a breakdown of possible outcomes.

Clozapine-resistant schizophrenia: clinical features, pathophysiology, and treatment

In moving to the literature specific to CRS, the greatest limitation at present is the lack of research specific to this population. To date, almost all our efforts have been clinically driven; this is a sizeable population and the lack of effective interventions available represents one of the greatest unmet needs in the current treatment of schizophrenia. There is a sizeable literature looking at alternatives to clozapine or for clozapine augmentation, but even this work is compromised since most of these studies have failed to utilize the developed criteria. Suboptimal clozapine response represents the common denominator in studies of this sort, but how this is defined varies between investigations. Beyond treatment, virtually no work has been done on better understanding CRS, a point that is clearly evident in the sections that follow.

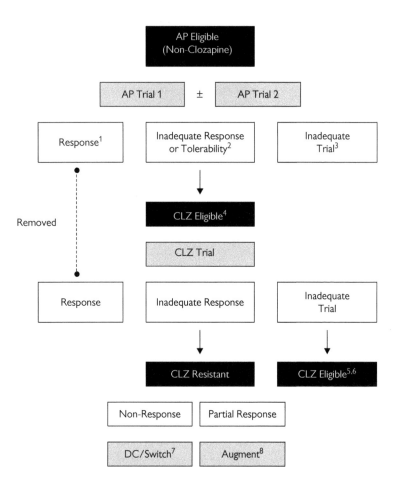

Fig. 12.1 The role of clozapine in the antipsychotic treatment of schizophrenia. AP, Antipsychotic; CLZ, clozapine.

[1]Various criteria have been proposed to define response/inadequate response using non-clozapine antipsychotics (see section on 'Criteria').

[2]Both inadequate antipsychotic (non-clozapine) response and intolerability to non-clozapine antipsychotics permit individuals to be designated clozapine-eligible.

[3]Inadequate response may represent suboptimal response to a particular drug, but may also result from an inadequate trial (i.e. inadequate antipsychotic dose or duration), in addition to other factors such as non-adherence, comorbid substance abuse, etc.

[4]A number of clozapine-eligible patients may not undertake such a trial; they may not be offered such a trial, or be excluded for other reasons (e.g. medical).

[5]Individuals may have been exposed to different antipsychotic trials, but for reasons detailed in (3), such as inadequate trials, they may still be clozapine-eligible.

[6]Similarly, reasons detailed in (3) can result in clozapine-eligible individuals continuing to remain clozapine-eligible despite being tried on clozapine (e.g. clozapine non-adherence, comorbid substance abuse).

[7]In individuals where there is no evidence of even suboptimal clinical response with clozapine, consideration should be given as to whether it should be continued.

[8]Given clozapine's position as antipsychotic of 'last resort' in treatment algorithms, partial or suboptimal response raises the question of augmentation strategies; however, limitations of such strategies are detailed in the text.

Clinical features

Refractory positive symptoms are central to CRS (Lee et al., 2015b; Mouaffak et al., 2006), and their prominence can obfuscate informed conclusions regarding other symptom domains (e.g. cognitive, negative). This said, one small study noted that neurocognition is impaired in both clozapine-responsive and -resistant individuals when compared to a group who responded to first-line antipsychotic treatment, but no differences were observed between the clozapine-responsive and -resistant samples (Anderson et al., 2015b). In line with this, it has been noted that, while clozapine can markedly impact refractory positive symptoms, effective clinical response does not necessarily translate to parallel improvements in measures of functional outcome (Lee et al., 2015a).

As noted, it has been estimated that somewhere between 12% and 20% of individuals with schizophrenia constitute CRS (Siskind et al., 2017). Evidence would suggest that the majority of these individuals have a form of treatment resistance that is evident from illness outset (Agid et al., 2011; Demjaha et al., 2017; Lally et al., 2016a). This said, findings also indicate that delayed clozapine use in individuals with TRS compromises response, suggesting that one can also evolve into CRS (Ucok et al., 2015; Yada et al., 2015; Yoshimura et al., 2017).

Further to this last point, numerous studies have attempted to delineate factors, both clinical and biological, associated with clozapine response versus nonresponse. These are not studies that have directly compared clozapine-responsive and -resistant populations, but instead focus on isolating the clozapine-responsive population. It is beyond the scope of this chapter to review these numerous lines of investigation and the reader is referred to the most recent review of this topic, which concluded that no factors have been identified that are unequivocally associated with clinical response (Suzuki et al., 2011). This same conclusion has been drawn in more focused reviews; for example, the pharmacogenetics of clozapine response (Kohlrausch, 2013; Sriretnakumar et al., 2015). Given the heterogeneity of schizophrenia, it is not surprising that there is a call for strategies that capture much more data in models of prediction (Lin et al., 2008; Semiz et al., 2007).

Pathophysiology

A small number of studies have focused on directly comparing clozapine responders and non-responders, with the caveat that definitions vary from one study to the next and only a very few have actually incorporated proposed criteria for CRS. Using computed tomography (CT), an earlier study reported that clozapine non-responders showed increased prefrontal sulcal prominence versus responders, a finding observed for both positive and negative symptoms, leading the authors to conclude that clozapine's response depends on prefrontal cortical function (Friedman et al., 1991). These findings were corroborated shortly thereafter by a second group also using CT; other cortical regions were also implicated in this study, particularly the lateral temporal lobe (Honer et al., 1995). In contrast, a subsequent magnetic resonance imaging (MRI) investigation found a relationship between response and the anterior superior temporal lobe but in this case the findings were in the opposite direction. That is, volume loss was associated with improved response, leading the authors to conclude that clozapine is effective even in the face of significant brain dysmorphology (Lauriello et al., 1998). Three perfusion studies have also added to this line of investigation. Using single proton emission computed tomography and [^{99m}Tc]HMPAO (hexamethylpropyleneamine oxime), it was reported that clozapine responders demonstrated lower prefrontal perfusion than non-responders. This subgroup also had higher subcortical perfusion than healthy controls, a difference that diminished with clozapine administration (Molina Rodriguez et al., 1996). A second such study reported that, when compared to clozapine non-responders, responders exhibited higher thalamic, basal ganglia, and prefrontal perfusion while on classical antipsychotics; further, subcortical and prefrontal activity decreased with clozapine (Molina Rodriguez et al., 1997). The final study by this same group did not dichotomize clozapine response and non-response, but instead evaluated clinical change across various dimensions (Molina et al., 2003). In addition, this study employed MRI and 18F-deoxyglucose positron emission tomography. Notably, results varied as a function of symptom domain; in the case of positive symptoms, though, there was a significant direct association with temporal cortex volume and an inverse association with dorsolateral prefrontal cortex cerebrospinal fluid.

Considerable work has focused on the role of glutamate in TRS (de Bartolomeis et al., 2012; Mouchlianitis et al., 2016; Nakajima et al., 2015; Taylor et al., 2017), a line of thinking that has extended to CRS as well. Again, evidence is nominal but a recent report involving magnetic resonance spectroscopy noted that first-line responders had higher dorsolateral prefrontal cortex total glutamate + glutamine levels scaled to creatine than those with CRS, while individuals with TRS had higher total glutamate + glutamine levels scaled to creatine in the putamen than the first-line responders as well as those with CRS (Goldstein et al., 2015). A second imaging study, in this case MRI, reported that clozapine-responsive and -resistant patients each differed from first-line responders in terms of reduced grey matter volume, although no significant volume differences were observed between each other (Anderson et al., 2015a).

Three genetic studies that employed criteria for CRS have been published. One report noted no association with the multidrug-resistant transporter 1 (*MDR1*) gene rs1045642 variant, which has been implicated in antipsychotic response (Mouaffak et al., 2011c). A second study investigated 15 genetic variants related to uncoupling proteins (UCP2, UCP4, UCP5), which play a role in neuroprotection and, again, have been implicated in schizophrenia. Compared to antipsychotic responders, the CRS sample demonstrated no differences in distribution of the respective alleles, although one haplotype spanning UCP4 was significantly underrepresented in the CRS population (Mouaffak et al., 2011a). The third investigation drew upon evidence that has implicated three common missense variants of the *DISC1* gene in schizophrenia: rs3738401 (Q264R), rs6675281

(L607F), and rs821616 (S704C). Once more, those with CRS were compared to antipsychotic responders, as well as normal controls, and a significant association between rs3738401 and CRS was noted (Mouaffak et al., 2011b).

Treatment

It has been proposed that treatment response defines at least three types of illness from a pathophysiological standpoint: (1) those who respond to non-clozapine antipsychotics; (2) those who are eligible for, and respond to, clozapine (CES); and (3) those who are clozapine-resistant (CRS) (Farooq et al., 2013; Lee et al., 2015b). In addition, it is possible that there is more than one subgroup in CRS; without effective treatments as well as clear mechanistic models, however, we can only conceptualize these as a single group for the time being.

Not surprisingly, there is a substantial body of evidence related to augmentation strategies in CRS, keeping in mind that this work really only gained momentum following the reintroduction of clozapine in different countries, including the USA, in the 1990s. This is reflected in Table 12.2, which provides an overview of 13 meta-analyses specific to this topic (Galling et al., 2017; Lally et al., 2016b; Paton et al., 2007; Porcelli et al., 2012; Sommer et al., 2012; Srisurapanont et al., 2015; Taylor and Smith, 2009; Taylor et al., 2012; Tiihonen et al., 2009; Veerman et al., 2014a; 2014b; Wang et al., 2010; Zheng et al., 2017). Of note, only findings related to randomized controlled trials (RCTs) are reviewed, and the results discussed here centre around improvement in total or positive symptoms rather than negative symptoms or tolerability. Positive findings are not discussed if current data are confined to single RCTs.

A number of different strategies have been investigated, including antipsychotics, antidepressants, mood stabilizers, glutamate modulators, and a cluster of other agents that have been captured in several of these meta-analyses, including ethyl-eicosapentaenoic acid (E-EPA), modafinil, memantine, and ginkgo biloba (Porcelli et al., 2012; Veerman et al., 2014a). Findings may be best summarized as follows:

i. Meta-analytic studies to date have evaluated a number of different strategies, although, collectively, substantive evidence strongly supporting a particular intervention remains lacking.

ii. A robust effect with electroconvulsive therapy (ECT) has been noted, but this meta-analysis was confined to one RCT and three open trials (Lally et al., 2016b).

iii. Findings for different strategies have varied between meta-analyses; this is evident, for example, with antiepileptic agents such as topiramate and lamotrigine (Porcelli et al., 2012; Sommer et al., 2012; Tiihonen et al., 2009; Zheng et al., 2017).

iv. Where favourable findings have been reported, the magnitude of change is frequently modest and of questionable clinical significance (Paton et al., 2007; Taylor and Smith, 2009; Taylor et al., 2012).

Table 12.2 Summary of findings from meta-analyses specific to augmentation strategies in clozapine-resistant schizophrenia

Strategy/reference (year)	Trials	Symptom outcome measures	Conclusions	Comments
Multiple strategies				
Veerman et al. (2014a)[1]				
Various antipsychotics	11 double-blind, placebo controlled RCTs (SGA 9, FGA 2, n=599)	Total, positive, negative, affective symptoms	No difference versus placebo	Outlier studies were removed in this report
Various antidepressants	Four double-blind, placebo controlled RCTs (n=111)	Total, positive, negative, affective symptoms	No difference versus placebo	
Sommer et al. (2014a)				
15 augmentation strategies forming four groups: Antiepileptics	Double-blind, placebo-controlled RCTs	Total symptom score; positive and negative symptoms	Significant results confined to agents represented by a single study.	Outlier studies were removed in this report
	8 (n=189)			
Antidepressants	4 (n=129)			
Antipsychotics	10 (n=548)			
Glutamatergics	7 (n=137)			
Porcelli et al. (2011)	Use of both RCTs and open studies. Meta-analysis confined to eight placebo-controlled RCTs with response data: risperidone (5); lamotrigine (3)	Global improvement	Both risperidone and lamotrigine showed no difference versus placebo	This report was subsequently challenged for missing RCTs in the case of lamotrigine, as well as mixing RCTs with lower quality evidence (Tiihonen et al., 2009)
62 augmentation studies forming five groups:				
Antipsychotics				
Antidepressants				
Mood stabilizers				
ECT				
Other[1]				

Antipsychotics

Various Antipsychotics

Galling et al. (2017)	31 RCTs (14 involving CLZ augmentation, 12 SGA, 2 FGA, n=612),	Total symptom reduction; study defined treatment response	No difference in both CLZ and non-CLZ studies	Studies broken down into 'high' and 'low' quality. Differences found only in low-quality and open studies
Taylor et al. (2012)	14 placebo-controlled RCTs (11 SGA, 3 FGA, n=734),		Small benefit	Also noted no benefit to trials >6 weeks (range 6–24 weeks)
Taylor and Smith (2009)	10 placebo-controlled RCTs (8 SGA, 2 FGA, n=522).	Total symptom reduction	Marginal benefit of doubtful clinical significance	Trial duration was not associated with outcome (range 6–16 weeks) Results supported by a further eight open studies reviewed
Paton et al. (2007)	4 placebo-controlled RCTs (4 SGA, n=166),	Total symptom reduction; response as defined by >20% decrease in total score	Weak evidence of therapeutic benefit	Studies >10 weeks showed a significant, albeit marginal, advantage

Specific antipsychotics

Aripiprazole

Srisurapanont et al. (2015)	4 RCTs (3, compared to placebo; 1, compared to haloperidol, n=347),	Total symptom reduction	Only trends for benefits on total and individual symptom scores	Patients' response to CLZ 'unsatisfactory' or 'not fully responsive + evidence of 'cardiometabolic risk'

Sulpiride

Wang et al. (2010)	4 RCTs (n=221)	Total symptom reduction, as well as individual symptom domains (positive, negative) Global score reduction	Short-term data (<12 weeks) showed a difference favouring augmentation that was non-significant. Longer term data showed no such difference	The study population for three of the four studies represented patients whose prominent symptoms were negative' Further, in the augmentation group, sulpiride was added from the outset. In the fourth study, which was 3 years in duration and focused on clozapine partial responders, improvement was reported in both positive and negative symptoms; however, this was an open study

continued >

Strategy/reference (year)	Trials	Symptom outcome measures	Conclusions	Comments
Antiepileptics				
Various antiepileptics				
Zheng et al. (2017)	22 RCTs (n=1227): topiramate (5, n=270), lamotrigine (8, n=299), sodium valproate (6, n=430); magnesium valproate (3, n=228)	Total symptom reduction; positive, negative, general psychopathology symptoms; response or remission	Significant improvement in positive and general symptom severity with topiramate and sodium valproate. Topiramate also showed improvement with negative symptoms, but was also associated with greater all-cause discontinuation	Outlier studies were removed in this report
Topiramate				
Lamotrigine				
Sodium valproate				
Magnesium valproate				
Specific antiepileptics				
Tiihonen et al. (2009)	5 double-blind, placebo-controlled RCTs (n=161), 10–24 weeks in duration	Total symptom reduction/response; positive and negative symptoms	Lamotrigine superior to placebo on each of these outcomes	Response, NNT = 4
Glutamate modulators				
Veerman et al. (2014b)	Double-blind, placebo controlled RCTs: glycine (3, n=57); topiramate (4, n=152); lamotrigine (6, n=185)	Total symptom reduction; positive and negative symptoms	Glycine significantly worsened positive symptoms and was not significantly different from placebo on total and negative symptoms. Topiramate and lamotrigine were not different from placebo on all three measures	Insufficient data regarding memantine, a voltage-dependent NMDA receptor antagonist
Glycine				
Topiramate				
Lamotrogine				

ECT

Lally et al. (2016b)	One single-blind RCT (n=39) + four open trials (n=32)	Response rate, as measured by predefined score reduction	Overall pooled proportion of response to CLZ + ECT = 54%	Use of open trials; while single-blind, the response rate in the RCT was 50%

[1]Single double-blind, placebo-controlled studies are reported for lithium and gingko biloba, as are two trials involving ethyl-eicosapentaenoic acid (E-EPA).

[2]Other: glycine, D-cycloserine, D-serine, ampakine CX-516, N-methylglycine, modafinil, memantine, mazindol, E-EPA.

CLZ, Clozapine; ECT, electroconvulsive therapy; FGA, first-generation antipsychotic; NMDA, N-methyl-D-aspartate; NNT, number needed to treat; RCT, randomized controlled trial; SGA, second-generation antipsychotic.

    v. Reports of clinical worsening have been reported (e.g. glycine and positive symptoms) (Veerman et al., 2014b).

Taken together, a number of different strategies have largely been negative and, where signals have been identified (e.g. with antiepileptics and ECT), the evidence is either conflicting or insufficient. Indeed, recently published guidelines opted to decline treatment recommendations for the psychotic features of CRS based on existing evidence (Remington et al., 2017). In pursuing effective treatment options, it will be important that we heed what does not work as well as what holds promise. For want of better, we unfortunately cling to strategies that are, simply put, without evidence.

Conclusion

URS or CRS owes its origin to the discovery of clozapine's unique efficacy in TRS, although current evidence suggests this occurs in only about 40% of cases (Siskind et al., 2017). The number of those who remain treatment-resistant is, however, artificially inflated by a further subgroup, also substantial in number, made up of individuals not offered a trial of clozapine or who decline it (Remington et al., 2016). Acknowledging schizophrenia's heterogeneity, it has been proposed that different subtypes can be elucidated based on clinical response (Farooq et al., 2013; Lee et al., 2015b). To do this, though, it is essential that we distinguish these different populations. Those who fail an adequate trial of clozapine are clearly different pathophysiologically from those responsive to clozapine but, until individuals are afforded such a trial, it is impossible to make such a distinction. This becomes critical as we seek treatments that specifically address the different subtypes, a point that, to date, has not been adequately embraced in study designs. Many investigations seeking to define markers or effective interventions for 'treatment resistance' have drawn upon mixed samples, compromising any reported results. Further, almost all studies currently published on the topic have failed to embrace established criteria in defining URS or CRS, and any interpretation of the existing evidence must take this into account.

    In terms of research on CRS going forward, we suggest a number of recommendations:

    i. To best define this population, we must accurately identify those individuals who have CRS, distinguishing them from those who have not received clozapine or had an adequate trial (Lee et al., 2015b; Remington et al., 2016).

    ii. Standardized criteria for CRS should be employed for diagnosis and treatment response (Lee et al., 2015b; Mouaffak et al., 2006; Remington et al., 2016).

iii. While treatment resistance can characterize different symptom domains related to schizophrenia, positive symptoms remain central, whether it is TRS or URS (Lee et al., 2015b; Mouaffak et al., 2006; Remington et al., 2016).

iv. Further to the previous point, functional status should not be part of criteria for defining CRS or response to interventions. Clinical recovery, as characterized by resolution of positive symptoms, does not necessarily translate to functional recovery (Lee et al., 2014).

v. We caution against the notion of a single intervention/treatment. Just as schizophrenia is heterogeneous, it is multidimensional, and research strategies are needed that focus on other symptom domains (e.g. those that seem more related to functioning—negative and cognitive) or other clinical features (e.g. aggression, mood). In fact, such a strategy better reflects changes captured in *The Diagnostic and Statistical Manual of Mental Disorders* (DSM-5), as well as the notion of personalized medicine, where an individual's treatment may be multidimensional and shaped by their specific profile across different domains (American Psychiatric Association, 2013).

vi. While we may assume that CRS is a single entity, this may not be the case (Farooq et al., 2013; Lee et al., 2015b).

Work specific to this population is in its earliest stages, not unlike the period that set the stage for clearly defined TRS criteria and the identification of clozapine's unique role in these individuals. Notably, TRS criteria were modified over time in the face of increased knowledge, and we should anticipate the same with current criteria for CRS. This said, we must work with what we have and begin the process of ensuring we accurately identify those individuals with CRS. With this as a foundation, we can then begin to build a systematic body of work spanning aetiology/pathophysiology, treatment, and outcome.

REFERENCES

Agid, O., Arenovich, T., Sajeev, G., et al. (2011). An algorithm-based approach to first-episode schizophrenia: response rates over 3 prospective antipsychotic trials with a retrospective data analysis. *J Clin Psychiatry*, 72, 1439–44.

American Psychiatric Association. (2013). *Diagnostic and Statistical Manual of Mental Disorders, Fifth Edition (DSM-V)*. Washington: American Psychiatric Publishing.

Anderson, V. M., Goldstein, M. E., Kydd, R. R., Russell, B. R. (2015a). Extensive grey matter volume reduction in treatment-resistant schizophrenia. *Int J Neuropsychopharmacol*, 18, 1–10.

Anderson, V. M., McIlwain, M. E., Kydd, R. R., Russell, B. R. (2015b). Does cognitive impairment in treatment-resistant and ultra-treatment-resistant schizophrenia differ from that in treatment responders? *Psychiatry Res*, 230, 811–18.

Baldessarini, R. J., Cohen, B. M., Teicher, M. H. (1988). Significance of neuroleptic dose and plasma level in the pharmacological treatment of psychoses. *Arch Gen Psychiatry*, 45, 79–91.

Bollini, P., Pampallona, S., Orza, M. J., Adams, M. E., Chalmers, T. C. (1994). Antipsychotic drugs: is more worse? A meta-analysis of the published randomized control trials. *Psychol Med*, 24, 307–16.

Brenner, H. D., Dencker, S. J., Goldstein, M. J., et al. (1990). Defining treatment refractoriness in schizophrenia. *Schizophr Bull*, 16, 551–61.

Conley, R. R., Buchanan, R. W. (1997). Evaluation of treatment-resistant schizophrenia. *Schizophr Bull*, 23, 663–74.

Davis, J. M., Chen, N. (2004). Dose response and dose equivalence of antipsychotics. *J Clin Psychopharmacol*, 24, 192–208.

De Bartolomeis, A., Sarappa, C., Magara, S., Iasevoli, F. (2012). Targeting glutamate system for novel antipsychotic approaches: relevance for residual psychotic symptoms and treatment resistant schizophrenia. *Eur J Pharmacol*, 682, 1–11.

Demjaha, A., Lappin, J. M., Stahl, D., et al. (2017). Antipsychotic treatment resistance in first-episode psychosis: prevalence, subtypes and predictors. *Psychol Med*, 47, 1981–9.

Dold, M., Leucht, S. (2014). Pharmacotherapy of treatment-resistant schizophrenia: a clinical perspective. *Evid Based Ment Health*, 17, 32–7.

Englisch, S., Zink, M. (2012). Treatment-resistant schizophrenia: evidence-based strategies. *Mens Sana Monogr*, 10, 20–32.

Farooq, S., Agid, O., Foussias, G., Remington, G. (2013). Using treatment response to subtype schizophrenia: proposal for a new paradigm in classification. *Schizophr Bull*, 39, 1169–72.

Friedman, L., Knutson, L., Shurell, M., Meltzer, H. Y. (1991). Prefrontal sulcal prominence is inversely related to response to clozapine in schizophrenia. *Biol Psychiatry*, 29, 865–77.

Fusar-Poli, P., Papanastasiou, E., Stahl, D., et al. (2015). Treatments of negative symptoms in schizophrenia: meta-analysis of 168 randomized placebo-controlled trials. *Schizophr Bull*, 41, 892–9.

Galling, B., Roldan, A., Hagi, K., et al. (2017). Antipsychotic augmentation vs. monotherapy in schizophrenia: systematic review, meta-analysis and meta-regression analysis. *World Psychiatry*, 16, 77–89.

Goldstein, M. E., Anderson, V. M., Pillai, A., Kydd, R. R., Russell, B. R. (2015). Glutamatergic neurometabolites in clozapine-responsive and -resistant schizophrenia. *Int J Neuropsychopharmacol*, 18, 1–9.

Guitton, C., Kinowski, J. M., Abbar, M., Chabrand, P., Bressolle, F. (1999). Clozapine and metabolite concentrations during treatment of patients with chronic schizophrenia. *J Clin Pharmacol*, 39, 721–8.

Hagan, J. J., Jones, D. N. (2005). Predicting drug efficacy for cognitive deficits in schizophrenia. *Schizophr Bull*, 31, 830–53.

Honer, W. G., Smith, G. N., LaPointe, J. S., MacEwan, G. W., Kopala, L., Altman, S. (1995). Regional cortical anatomy and clozapine response in refractory schizophrenia. *Neuropsychopharmacology*, 13, 85–7.

Itil, T. M., Keskiner, A., Fink, M. (1966). Therapeutic studies in 'therapy resistant' schizophrenic patients. *Compr Psychiatry*, 7, 488–93.

Kane, J., Honigfeld, G., Singer, J., Meltzer, H. (1988). Clozapine for the treatment-resistant schizophrenic. A double-blind comparison with chlorpromazine. *Arch Gen Psychiatry*, 45, 789–96.

Kapur, S., Zipursky, R. B., Remington, G. (1999). Clinical and theoretical implications of 5-HT2 and D2 receptor occupancy of clozapine, risperidone, and olanzapine in schizophrenia. *Am J Psychiatry*, 156, 286–93.

Kapur, S., Zipursky, R., Jones, C., Remington, G., Houle, S. (2000). Relationship between dopamine D(2) occupancy, clinical response, and side effects: a double-blind PET study of first-episode schizophrenia. *Am J Psychiatry*, 157, 514–20.

Kohlrausch, F. B. (2013). Pharmacogenetics in schizophrenia: a review of clozapine studies. *Rev Bras Psiquiatr*, 35, 305–17.

Kristensen, D., Hageman, I., Bauer, J., Jorgensen, M. B., Correll, C. U. (2013). Antipsychotic polypharmacy in a treatment-refractory schizophrenia population receiving adjunctive treatment with electroconvulsive therapy. *J ECT*, 29, 271–6.

Lally, J., Ajnakina, O., Di Forti, M., et al. (2016a). Two distinct patterns of treatment resistance: clinical predictors of treatment resistance in first-episode schizophrenia spectrum psychoses. *Psychol Med*, 46, 3231–40.

Lally, J., Tully, J., Robertson, D., Stubbs, B., Gaughran, F., MacCabe, J. H. (2016b). Augmentation of clozapine with electroconvulsive therapy in treatment resistant schizophrenia: a systematic review and meta-analysis. *Schizophr Res*, 171, 219–24.

Lauriello, J., Mathalon, D. H., Rosenbloom, M., et al. (1998). Association between regional brain volumes and clozapine response in schizophrenia. *Biol Psychiatry*, 43, 879–86.

Lee, J., Takeuchi, H., Fervaha, G., Bhaloo, A., Powell, V., Remington, G. (2014). Relationship between clinical improvement and functional gains with clozapine in schizophrenia. *Eur Neuropsychopharmacol*, 24, 1622–9.

Lee, J., Fervaha, G., Takeuchi, H., Powell, V., Remington, G. (2015a). Positive symptoms are associated with clinicians' global impression in treatment-resistant schizophrenia. *J Clin Psychopharmacol*, 35, 237–41.

Lee, J., Takeuchi, H., Fervaha, G., et al. (2015b). Subtyping schizophrenia by treatment response: antipsychotic development and the central role of positive symptoms. *Can J Psychiatry*, 60, 515–22.

Lee, J., Bies, R., Takeuchi, H., et al. (2016). Quantifying intraindividual variations in plasma clozapine levels: a population pharmacokinetic approach. *J Clin Psychiatry*, 77, 681–7.

Lin, C. C., Wang, Y. C., Chen, J. Y., et al. (2008). Artificial neural network prediction of clozapine response with combined pharmacogenetic and clinical data. *Comput Methods Programs Biomed*, 91, 91–9.

Marder, S. R. (2006). Drug initiatives to improve cognitive function. *J Clin Psychiatry*, 67 (Suppl. 9), 31–5; discussion 36–42.

Miyamoto, S., Jarskog, L. F., Fleischhacker, W. W. (2014). New therapeutic approaches for treatment-resistant schizophrenia: a look to the future. *J Psychiatr Res*, 58, 1–6.

Molina, V., Reig, S., Sarramea, F., et al. (2003). Anatomical and functional brain variables associated with clozapine response in treatment-resistant schizophrenia. *Psychiatry Res*, 124, 153–61.

Molina Rodriguez, V., Montz Andree, R., Perez Castejon, M. J., Capdevila Garcia, E., Carreras Delgado, J. L., Rubia Vila, F. J. (1996). SPECT study of regional cerebral perfusion in neuroleptic-resistant schizophrenic patients who responded or did not respond to clozapine. *Am J Psychiatry*, 153, 1343–6.

Molina Rodriguez, V., Montz Andree, R., Perez Castejon, M. J., et al. (1997). Cerebral perfusion correlates of negative symptomatology and parkinsonism in a sample of treatment-refractory schizophrenics: an exploratory 99mTc-HMPAO SPET study. *Schizophr Res*, 25, 11–20.

Mouaffak, F., Tranulis, C., Gourevitch, R., et al. (2006). Augmentation strategies of clozapine with antipsychotics in the treatment of ultraresistant schizophrenia. *Clin Neuropharmacol*, 29, 28–33.

Mouaffak, F., Kebir, O., Bellon, A., et al. (2011a). Association of an UCP4 (SLC25A27) haplotype with ultra-resistant schizophrenia. *Pharmacogenomics*, 12, 185–93.

Mouaffak, F., Kebir, O., Chayet, M., et al. (2011b). Association of Disrupted in Schizophrenia 1 (DISC1) missense variants with ultra-resistant schizophrenia. *Pharmacogenomics J*, 11, 267–73.

Mouaffak, F., Kebir, O., Picard, V., et al. (2011c). Ultra-resistant schizophrenia is not associated with the multidrug-resistant transporter 1 (MDR1) gene rs1045642 variant. *J Clin Psychopharmacol*, 31, 236–8.

Mouchlianitis, E., Mccutcheon, R., Howes, O. D. (2016). Brain-imaging studies of treatment-resistant schizophrenia: a systematic review. *Lancet Psychiatry*, 3, 451–63.

Nakajima, S., Takeuchi, H., Plitman, E., et al. (2015). Neuroimaging findings in treatment-resistant schizophrenia: a systematic review: lack of neuroimaging correlates of treatment-resistant schizophrenia. *Schizophr Res*, 164, 164–75.

Nielsen, R. E., Levander, S., Kjaersdam Telleus, G., et al. (2015). Second-generation antipsychotic effect on cognition in patients with schizophrenia—a meta-analysis of randomized clinical trials. *Acta Psychiatr Scand*, 131, 185–96.

Paton, C., Whittington, C., Barnes, T. R. (2007). Augmentation with a second antipsychotic in patients with schizophrenia who partially respond to clozapine: a meta-analysis. *J Clin Psychopharmacol*, 27, 198–204.

Porcelli, S., Balzarro, B., Serretti, A. (2012). Clozapine resistance: augmentation strategies. *Eur Neuropsychopharmacol*, 22, 165–82.

Remington, G. (2003). Understanding antipsychotic 'atypicality': a clinical and pharmacological moving target. *J Psychiatry Neurosci*, 28, 275–84.

Remington, G., Foussias, G., Agid, O., Takeuchi, T., Rao, N. (2012). Anti-schizophrenia drugs: the next generation. *JPPS*, 9, 49–52.

Remington, G., Lee, J., Agid, O., et al. (2016). Clozapine's critical role in treatment resistant schizophrenia: ensuring both safety and use. *Expert Opin Drug Saf*, 15, 1193–203.

Remington, G., Addington, D., Honer, W., Ismail, Z., Raedler, T., Teehan, M. (2017). Guidelines for the pharmacotherapy of schizophrenia in adults. *Can J Psychiatry*, 62, 604–16.

Rubio, J. M., Correll, C. U. (2017). Duration and relevance of untreated psychiatric disorders, 1: psychotic disorders. *J Clin Psychiatry*, 78, 358–9.

Samara, M. T., Dold, M., Gianatsi, M., et al. (2016). Efficacy, acceptability, and tolerability of antipsychotics in treatment-resistant schizophrenia: a network meta-analysis. *JAMA Psychiatry*, 73, 199–210.

CHAPTER 12

Semiz, U. B., Cetin, M., Basoglu, C., et al. (2007). Clinical predictors of therapeutic response to clozapine in a sample of Turkish patients with treatment-resistant schizophrenia. *Prog Neuropsychopharmacol Biol Psychiatry*, 31, 1330–6.

Siskind, D., Siskind, V., Kisely, S. (2017). Clozapine response rates among people with treatment-resistant schizophrenia: data from a systematic review and meta-analysis. *Can J Psychiatry*, 62, 772–7.

Sommer, I. E., Begemann, M. J., Temmerman, A., Leucht, S. (2012). Pharmacological augmentation strategies for schizophrenia patients with insufficient response to clozapine: a quantitative literature review. *Schizophr Bull*, 38, 1003–11.

Sriretnakumar, V., Huang, E., Muller, D. J. (2015). Pharmacogenetics of clozapine treatment response and side-effects in schizophrenia: an update. *Expert Opin Drug Metab Toxicol*, 11, 1709–31.

Srisurapanont, M., Suttajit, S., Maneeton, N., Maneeton, B. (2015). Efficacy and safety of aripiprazole augmentation of clozapine in schizophrenia: a systematic review and meta-analysis of randomized-controlled trials. *J Psychiatr Res*, 62, 38–47.

Subramanian, S., Vollm, B. A., Huband, N. (2017). Clozapine dose for schizophrenia. *Cochrane Database Syst Rev*, 6, CD009555.

Suzuki, T., Remington, G., Mulsant, B. H., et al. (2011). Treatment resistant schizophrenia and response to antipsychotics: a review. *Schizophr Res*, 133, 54–62.

Suzuki, T., Remington, G., Mulsant, B. H., et al. (2012). Defining treatment-resistant schizophrenia and response to antipsychotics: a review and recommendation. *Psychiatry Res*, 197, 1–6.

Taylor, D. L., Tiwari, A. K., Lieberman, J. A., et al. (2017). Pharmacogenetic analysis of functional glutamate system gene variants and clinical response to clozapine. *Mol Neuropsychiatry*, 2, 185–97.

Taylor, D. M., Smith, L. (2009). Augmentation of clozapine with a second antipsychotic—a meta-analysis of randomized, placebo-controlled studies. *Acta Psychiatr Scand*, 119, 419–25.

Taylor, D. M., Smith, L., Gee, S. H., Nielsen, J. (2012). Augmentation of clozapine with a second antipsychotic—a meta-analysis. *Acta Psychiatr Scand*, 125, 15–24.

Tiihonen, J., Wahlbeck, K., Kiviniemi, V. (2009). The efficacy of lamotrigine in clozapine-resistant schizophrenia: a systematic review and meta-analysis. *Schizophr Res*, 109, 10–14.

Ucok, A., Cikrikcili, U., Karabulut, S., et al. (2015). Delayed initiation of clozapine may be related to poor response in treatment-resistant schizophrenia. *Int Clin Psychopharmacol*, 30, 290–5.

Veerman, S. R., Schulte, P. F., Begemann, M. J., De Haan, L. (2014a). Non-glutamatergic clozapine augmentation strategies: a review and meta-analysis. *Pharmacopsychiatry*, 47, 231–8.

Veerman, S. R., Schulte, P. F., Begemann, M. J., Engelsbel, F., De Haan, L. (2014b). Clozapine augmented with glutamate modulators in refractory schizophrenia: a review and metaanalysis. *Pharmacopsychiatry*, 47, 185–94.

Wang, J., Omori, I. M., Fenton, M., Soares, B. (2010). Sulpiride augmentation for schizophrenia. *Cochrane Database Syst Rev*, CD008125.

Warnez, S., Alessi-Severini, S. (2014). Clozapine: a review of clinical practice guidelines and prescribing trends. *BMC Psychiatry*, 14, 102.

Williams, L., Newton, G., Roberts, K., Finlayson, S., Brabbins, C. (2002). Clozapine-resistant schizophrenia: a positive approach. *Br J Psychiatry*, 181, 184–7.

Yada, Y., Yoshimura, B., Kishi, Y. (2015). Correlation between delay in initiating clozapine and symptomatic improvement. *Schizophr Res*, 168, 585–6.

Yoshimura, B., Yada, Y., So, R., Takaki, M., Yamada, N. (2017). The critical treatment window of clozapine in treatment-resistant schizophrenia: secondary analysis of an observational study. *Psychiatry Res*, 250, 65–70.

Zheng, W., Xiang, Y. T., Yang, X. H., Xiang, Y. Q., De Leon, J. (2017). Clozapine augmentation with antiepileptic drugs for treatment-resistant schizophrenia: a meta-analysis of randomized controlled trials. *J Clin Psychiatry*, 78, e498–e505.

CHAPTER 12

Illustrative case studies

Ofer Agid, Thomas R. E. Barnes, Majella Byrne, Araba Chintoh, Christoph U. Correll, Siobhan Gee, Oliver Howes, Suzanne Jolley, John Kane, John Lally, Jimmy Lee, James H. MacCabe, Stephen Marder, Robert McCutcheon, Jimmi Nielsen, Emmanuelle Peters, Gary Remington, Christopher Rohde, Hiroyoshi Takeuchi, David Taylor, and Yvonne Yang

---

KEY POINTS

- These case studies illustrate key aspects of the treatment of schizophrenia and challenges seen in clinical practice.

- The art of clinical practice includes interpreting and applying evidence to help individual patients who often do not fit into the categories used in clinical trials.

- The cases show the application of evidence, and also its limitations, in real-world settings.

- The cases emphasize the need for the evidence and recommendations discussed throughout this book to be considered in the individual context of each patient.

Case 1: A case of treatment resistance evident from first presentation

John Lally and James H. MacCabe

Mr AB is a 30-year-old man with a history of schizophrenia, diagnosed when he was 19. He has a history of contact with psychiatric services dating from the age of 17.

His early developmental milestones and medical history were uneventful. He smoked cannabis from the age of 14, progressing to using ecstasy and amphetamines before stopping all substance use during his later teenage years. He was assessed by psychiatry services at the age of 17 owing to a period of social withdrawal and deteriorating school performance. He was diagnosed with depression and treated for 2 months with sertraline before discontinuing it. He completed school, failing several examinations, and not progressing to university like his older siblings. He then worked in several short-term employment positions, with a pattern of short-lived employment because of poor time-keeping.

He next presented to psychiatric services aged 19, when his parents, increasingly concerned by irritability and aggressive outbursts at home, encouraged him to attend. He had not worked for 6 months, and had become increasingly withdrawn and disconnected from his peer groups. His parents reported that they had been increasingly concerned about his mental health and behaviour for approximately 2 years. For a number of months he had become increasingly isolated and had become convinced that his parents were trying to control him and were able to influence his thinking. He believed that he had the power to control situations using his mind only. His isolative and intermittent aggressive behaviour was driven 'by paranoia' and intrusive 'psychotic symptoms'.

He was diagnosed with a first-episode schizophrenia and commenced risperidone. This was titrated to 6 mg daily and, despite reported adherence, led to partial response only. A further deterioration in mental state led to a first hospital admission under a compulsory admission order 4 months after risperidone initiation. He believed that others could control his thoughts and that he could hear people providing a running commentary on his actions, likening the experiences to hearing a universal voice. He reported that he had been the subject of invasive experiments by doctors and local police for the past 2 years. He believed that a transmission device was attached to his body and then internally inserted to monitor him. He reported that others could implant thoughts that were not his own into his mind. At hospitalization, he denied recent cannabis or other drug use, and his urinary drug screen was negative. He reported that he had stopped using cannabis over 1 year ago.

He was treated with olanzapine 20 mg daily, attaining plasma olanzapine levels of 40 µg/L (within the expected range), with only a partial response. Concerns remained about longer term treatment adherence, which led to a switch to flupentixol decanoate depot injection, titrated to 200 mg every 2 weeks. This was combined with olanzapine 10 mg daily and he was discharged from hospital. Psychotic symptoms persisted, and he required supportive care in the community, temporarily living in nursing supervised accommodation. He had four further compulsory hospital admissions over the next 5 years (each with durations of 3–6 months), with various antipsychotic combination strategies being implemented. Throughout, he remained guarded and displayed limited insight.

He was readmitted to hospital at the age of 25 after a period of increased paranoid symptomatology, focused on a belief that neighbours were acting malevolently towards him. There was evidence of self-neglect and he had lost a significant amount of weight. He had not worked for 6 years, and had never re-engaged with academic pursuits, with evidence of marked social isolation, having withdrawn from all contact with family and friends. There was no history of illicit substance use over this time.

He was commenced on clozapine, titrated to 450 mg daily, with plasma clozapine concentrations of 0.45 mg/L. He displayed a good response to clozapine, with symptom remission at 6 months. Subsequently, a comorbid depressive episode was diagnosed. This was treated with sertraline combined with cognitive behavioural therapy.

Learning points

- This case illustrates limited response to a series of non-clozapine antipsychotics, highlighting that treatment resistance is present from first presentation in a significant proportion of patients (see Chapter 4).
- Testing for plasma levels of antipsychotics and a trial of a long-acting injectable antipsychotic was used to rule out pseudo-treatment resistance in this case. These are important components of the evaluation of treatment resistance (see Chapter 2).
- In this case, clozapine was tried after more than 5 years of illness, by which time marked social and occupational impairment had developed. Careful assessment for treatment resistance, and appropriate, early use of clozapine should be considered early in the course of the illness (see Chapters 4 and 6).
- A younger age of illness onset, particularly before the age of 20, is a risk factor for treatment resistance (see Chapter 4).
- Treatment resistance is associated with significant functional decline, lost employment and educational opportunities, and a significant impact on health resources due to hospitalization and need for intensive community support (see Chapter 4).

Case 2: A case of early-onset treatment resistance

Robert McCutcheon, Christoph U. Correll, Oliver Howes, and John Kane

Ms Burroughs had experienced an episode of depression in her adolescence. This had been successfully treated, and she had not had any subsequent contact with mental health services prior to her first inpatient admission at the age of 33. This admission occurred following a 3-month decline in functioning. She had resigned from her job as a university lecturer, following experiences in which she believed messages in her students' essays were instructing her to travel to Africa as part of a spiritual mission. She was detained under the Mental Health Act after behaving bizarrely at an airport, and was then admitted to a psychiatric hospital.

She was initially treated with oral paliperidone, which was changed to long-acting injectable paliperidone after she consistently refused oral medication. After 4 months of treatment, there was a slight improvement in her symptoms and she was discharged to a community mental health team. Her delusional beliefs were less tenaciously held, but she continued to be distressed by auditory hallucinations and passivity phenomena, which disrupted her sleep and prevented her from returning to work. Owing to lack of a clinically meaningful benefit, the long-acting injectable paliperidone was stopped and she commenced treatment with oral amisulpride, which she took. However, this treatment did not show any significant benefit either. Pharmacy records and antipsychotic plasma levels indicated a good level of adherence. Clinical assessment using the Positive And Negative Syndrome Scale (PANSS) showed a positive symptom score of 21, a negative symptom score of 12, and a general symptom score of 23, with mod-erate–marked severity scores for hallucinations and delusion ratings. A diagnosis of early-onset treatment-resistant schizophrenia (positive symptom domain) was made. Functioning, as assessed by the global assessment of function (GAF), was 45, indicating moderate–severe functional impairment. Clozapine treatment was commenced 12 months following her initial episode and, at a dose of 350 mg per day (clozapine plasma level >0.35 μg/L), she noted a marked improvement in her sleep, and a noticeable reduction in the frequency and intensity of her auditory hallucinations. Her functioning continued to improve over the following 6 months and she was able to return to employment on a part-time basis. At a later follow-up appointment, her GAF was scored at 65 (indicating only mild impairment), and PANSS symptom ratings were all low (positive = 10, negative = 8, and gen-eral = 20), with no more than a mild rating on any individual item.

Learning points

- Treatment resistance can be apparent from illness onset (see Chapters 3 and 4).
- The use of long-acting injectable medication and antipsychotic plasma levels allows the clinical team to rule out covert non-adherence or inadequate plasma levels owing to other factors as a reason for insufficient response to two antipsychotics (see Chapter 3).
- Recording of both functioning and symptom scale scores allows subse-quent clinicians to have a more accurate measure of the patient's base-line clinical state and the effect of medication treatment and changes (see Chapter 3).

Case 3: A case of pseudo-treatment resistance

Robert McCutcheon, Christoph U. Correll, Oliver Howes, and John Kane

Mr Smith, a 25-year-old Caucasian male, was seen in an outpatient clinic with his mother for a routine 6-monthly appointment. A review of his clinical notes indicated that he had had his first psychotic episode at age 21 while a univer-sity student, and he had initially made a good recovery following treatment with risperidone. On assessment in the clinic, he was pleasant but vague in his an-swers, with a degree of thought disorder meaning that, at times, the meaning of his words was hard to grasp, and he frequently seemed distracted. He denied experiencing any psychotic symptoms and stated that he was happy with his current treatment. His mother, however, voiced concerns that Mr Smith had become increasingly withdrawn over the past 6 months, and that she frequently overheard him speaking to himself.

Antipsychotic treatment was changed to olanzapine on the basis that he appeared to be continuing to suffer from significant psychotic symptoms. There was limited change in Mr Smith's mental state, and it was felt that his illness might be treatment-resistant. At a subsequent appointment, however, antipsychotic plasma levels were found to be undetectable. When this was discussed with Mr Smith, he stated that he had stopped taking antipsychotics regularly 6 months ago, as he found it hard to remember to take medication. He was initially reluctant to consider a long-acting injectable antipsychotic, but agreed to a trial to determine if it had any benefit. Flupentixol decanoate i.m. was commenced and a noticeable improvement in Mr Smith's mental state was observed over the following 2 months. In particular, he appeared less distracted, and his mother noted that he became more sociable and returned to some of his previous interests.

Learning points

- Information from friends and family can be essential to a comprehensive assessment of treatment response or lack thereof. This is particularly the case when the clinician is unfamiliar with the patient or the patient is guarded or has limited illness insight (see Chapter 3).
- The use of antipsychotic plasma levels can provide valuable information regarding the adequacy of treatment, including indicating inadequate adherence (see Chapter 3).
- It is possible for non-adherence to be discussed in a collaborative fashion, and for solutions to be found with the patient (see Chapter 3).

Case 4: Case of treatment resistance with dramatic response to clozapine

Yvonne Yang and Stephen Marder

RR was a 54-year-old man who dropped out of university when he became psychotic at the age of 21. He responded poorly to antipsychotic medications and was hospitalized several times at a state hospital and resided in a locked facility between hospitalizations. Symptoms included suspicious delusions and aggressive behaviours. He was admitted to hospital in Los Angeles, USA, and started on clozapine in the early 1990s. Within a month of receiving clozapine he was symptom-free. Within 2 years he re-enrolled at university, graduated, and received his Masters in Education. He has taught in public school for more than 20 years since then, has friends, but never married. He is currently managed on 150 mg of clozapine at bedtime.

Learning points
- This case illustrates a severe, incapacitating illness with a poor response to first-line antipsychotic treatment from onset but a dramatic early improvement with clozapine (see Chapters 4 and 6).
- Response to clozapine can lead to remission and functional recovery that is sustained over many years (see Chapter 6).

Case 5: Case of treatment resistance with clozapine response and side effects

Yvonne Yang and Stephen Marder

RB is a 38-year-old woman from an Asian American family who developed psychotic symptoms while in high school. She developed persecutory delusions about a boyfriend as well as auditory hallucinations. Medication trials included aripiprazole, risperidone, and ziprasidone, but symptoms persisted despite adequate doses and assured adherence. After transitioning to clozapine her symptoms improved substantially. She is now able to attend a daycare programme and she often helps with the family business, which includes an ethnic deli. On 325 mg of clozapine she has nighttime drooling and she experienced a 15-pound weight gain. The family observes that she only experiences auditory hallucinations at night when she is alone in her room. At those times she is often heard talking to herself. She is no longer tormented by suspicious delusions.

Learning points
- This case illustrates poor response to a number of different first-line antipsychotics followed by a marked response to clozapine (see Chapter 5).
- Some residual symptoms persist despite clozapine treatment but are not distressing or impairing, and treatment has enabled her to regain some role functioning.
- Hypersalivation and weight gain are two of the most common side effects of clozapine. Management includes behavioural advice or, if this does not work, pharmacological options such as hyoscine for hypersalivation and metformin for weight gain (see Chapter 7).

Case 6: Case of a patient experiencing a seizure whilst taking clozapine

Christopher Rohde and Jimmi Nielsen

This is the case of a 35-year-old man diagnosed with paranoid schizophrenia. He was non-responsive to several antipsychotics but, during the past 2 years, was successfully treated with 450 mg clozapine per day. Suddenly, he developed pneumonia with a fever of 39°C and 2 days later he had a seizure. Previously there had been no history of seizures. Plasma levels of clozapine revealed a doubling relative to the last level prior to these problems and clozapine was paused for 2 days and then reinstated at 450 mg.

Learning points

• During infection clozapine levels may increase dramatically, which may trigger dose-dependent adverse effects such as seizures (see Chapter 7).

• Prophylactic antiepileptic treatment is not warranted after a single seizure, but the psychiatrist should ensure that dose adjustment occurs in case of new infections.

• In patients with seizures without any concomitant infection, treatment with lamotrigine or valproate is recommended. Electroencephalogram and computed tomography should be performed if the clinical features suggest that a cause other than clozapine is high on the differential diagnosis (see Chapter 7).

Case 7: Case of orthostatic hypotension on clozapine

Christopher Rohde and Jimmi Nielsen

This describes the case of a 48-year-old woman with disorganized schizophrenia. Clozapine was initiated because of poor response to previous antipsychotic drugs. During titration, she developed orthostatic hypotension when the clozapine dose reached 250 mg per day. The dose was reduced to 100 mg twice-daily and the orthostatic hypotension resolved but she had a psychotic relapse. After 3 weeks, the clozapine dose was increased to 100 + 0 + 0 + 150 mg again and she was advised to rise slowly from horizontal positions and to drink enough water to maintain blood pressure. As tachyphylaxis often occurs after a few weeks, this regimen was tried for 3 weeks. However, the orthostatic hypotension continued. The clozapine dosing was changed to 250 mg at bedtime to minimize daytime hypotension. Whilst changing the dosing regimen reduced the hypotension, this was not sufficient to prevent symptomatic hypotension. In view of this, compression socks were prescribed. Unfortunately, compliance with compression socks was low and this approach was not effective. In view of this a small dose of fludrocortisone acetate was prescribed instead. This alleviated the orthostatic hypotension and made it possible to continue the dose of 250 mg clozapine per day.

Learning points

• Orthostatic hypotension is common during treatment with clozapine and is mediated by antagonism of the alpha-1-noradrenergic receptor (see Chapter 7).

- As illustrated in the case, several treatment options exist (see Chapter 7). Be aware that other alpha-1-antagonists potentiate this adverse effect and, if possible, discontinue these medications.

Case 8: A case of rapid relapse on clozapine associated with smoking

Siobhan Gee and David Taylor

Miss A is a 36-year-old Caucasian patient who has been taking 125 mg clozapine twice-daily for treatment-resistant schizophrenia for the past 2 months. Clozapine was started during her current hospital admission and her illness is now sufficiently well treated to allow discharge back to supported accommodation. Miss A is very pleased to be discharged as she does not like her room on the ward, and because she hasn't been able to smoke as the hospital and grounds are non-smoking areas. She is discharged successfully but experiences a relapse in mental state after just 6 weeks. Her keyworker is certain that Miss A has been fully compliant with her clozapine as the staff in her accommodation have been supervising her doses. The junior doctor who admits her to hospital is not so sure, so he takes a plasma level. It is returned as being 0.15 µg/L. The doctor looks back through her notes from the last admission and sees that her clozapine plasma level before being discharged had been around 0.38 µg/L. The ward pharmacist completes a medication history for Miss A. She finds that Miss A usually smokes 40 cigarettes per day and is not very happy about being given nicotine replacement therapy again on this admission. The pharmacist points out that the change in smoking habit is likely to have contributed to the reduction in clozapine plasma level and subsequent relapse. Miss A is re-established on a therapeutic dose of clozapine, and responds quickly. She is discharged back to her community placement but this time the community psychiatric team are contacted and asked to monitor clozapine plasma levels weekly after discharge, as Miss A is not willing to stop smoking. They find that her clozapine plasma levels drop over the first 2 weeks of discharge from hospital. The community consultant psychiatrist increases her clozapine dose carefully, and after 6 weeks her plasma level is stable at 0.42 µg/L at a clozapine dose of 200 mg twice-daily, and she remains well.

Learning points

- There is good evidence that plasma levels of clozapine are linked to therapeutic response, and trough levels of at least 0.35 µg/L are generally considered as the minimum level for a therapeutic response (see Chapter 8).
- Cigarette smoking induces liver enzymes that metabolize clozapine, in particular cytochrome 1A, which increases the metabolism of clozapine and reduces plasma levels. Cigarette smokers generally require higher doses of clozapine as a result (see Chapter 8).

• Patients should be warned to let staff know about changes in smoking habits as these may have marked effects on plasma levels of clozapine.

Case 9: A case of benign ethnic neutropenia

Siobhan Gee and David Taylor

Mr B is a 27-year-old patient of African Caribbean ethnicity who was first diagnosed with schizophrenia aged 18. Since diagnosis he has received olanzapine up to 20 mg daily, which was ineffective, paliperidone depot 150 mg monthly, which caused extrapyramidal side effects and did not fully treat his positive symptoms, and sulpiride 1200 mg daily which was also ineffective. His illness was then felt to be treatment-resistant, and he was started on clozapine. After 3 weeks of treatment he was less thought-disordered and described his auditory hallucinations as reducing in frequency. However, his neutrophil count dropped from a baseline of around $2.0 \times 10^9/L$ to $1.6 \times 10^9/L$. Clozapine treatment was continued and the next blood draw taken 4 days later. The neutrophils were now $2.1 \times 10^9/L$. Weekly monitoring of the full blood count (FBC) was continued, and at week 5 neutrophil count was $1.3 \times 10^9/L$. Clozapine was stopped, and the next FBC (3 days later) showed the neutrophil count to be $1.9 \times 10^9/L$. Mr B was started on amisulpride 400 mg b.d., which was titrated up to 1.2 g b.d. over the course of the next month. Unfortunately, he became floridly psychotic despite this treatment. The multidisciplinary team and Mr B's family felt that his psychotic illness was more effectively treated with clozapine than with any other antipsychotic he had tried. A consultant haematologist was contacted for an opinion on the low neutrophil counts, which still remained in the range of $2.0 \times 10^9/L$ during the course of amisulpride treatment. The haematologist diagnosed Mr B with benign ethnic neutropenia (BEN) and advised the psychiatric team that she felt it unlikely that the low neutrophil levels were related to treatment with clozapine. Mr B was started on lithium carbonate, titrated to a plasma level of 0.4 µg/L. His baseline neutrophil counts rose to $2.5–3.0 \times 10^9/L$. The clozapine monitoring company was contacted and, with the diagnosis of BEN made by the haematologist, registered Mr B as having BEN and a lower range of reference values for his routine blood results was agreed. Mr B was re-started on clozapine in conjunction with lithium, and all subsequent neutrophil levels were in the range of $2.5–3.0 \times 10^9/L$.

Learning points

• Neutrophil counts need to be monitored during clozapine treatment because of the risk of agranulocytosis, and licensing regimes often require clozapine to be stopped if neutrophil levels fall below $1.5 \times 10^9/L$ as a result (see Chapter 6).

• A large number of people with African or Middle Eastern ancestry naturally have lower neutrophil counts than people with other ancestries, as is the case here where Mr B's neutrophil counts vary between 1.3 and 2.0 × 10^9/L. This does not put them at increased risk of clozapine-induced agranulocytosis and is termed benign ethnic neutropenia (BEN) (see Chapters 6 and 8).

• Where there is evidence that low neutrophil levels predated clozapine in people with African or Middle Eastern ancestry, a diagnosis of BEN may be considered. It is advisable to seek advice from a haematologist to exclude other causes of low neutrophils. The blood count cut-offs used in clozapine monitoring regimes can be lowered in cases of BEN (see Chapters 6 and 8).

• Lithium treatment can be used to increase neutrophil counts, although it does not prevent agranulocytosis (see Chapter 8).

Case 10: A case illustrating the use of high-dose and combination antipsychotic medication in treatment-resistant schizophrenia

Thomas R. E. Barnes

A 41-year-old female inpatient had a 15-year history of schizophrenia characterized by persistent delusions, usually of a persecutory or grandiose nature, and auditory hallucinations. The intensity of these psychotic symptoms had fluctuated markedly over the years and adversely affected her occupational and social functioning. Past treatment included trials of various antipsychotic medications, including aripiprazole, quetiapine, amisulpride, and risperidone, all of which had proved unsuccessful. However, her illness had responded well to clozapine treatment and she had returned to a high level of social competence and interpersonal functioning. The patient acknowledged that on clozapine she had been well, with 'no voices, no symptoms, no black magic'. However, clozapine had been discontinued because of cardiac symptoms. Subsequently, a high-dose antipsychotic medication regimen was initiated: flupentixol decanoate 400 mg i.m. every 2 weeks and oral aripiprazole 30 mg a day. On this regimen, there were no evident affective or negative symptoms, but she was again expressing a host of persecutory delusions and reporting persistent and disturbing auditory hallucinations. In terms of insight, while she accepted that she had a psychiatric illness that required treatment, she attributed many of her symptoms to black magic. Although the patient was well kempt, made good eye contact, engaged with psychosocial activities on the ward, and was apparently adherent to the high-dose antipsychotic treatment prescribed, the level of fluctuation in the severity of her psychotic symptoms and her preoccupation with them precluded discharge from hospital.

Learning points

This case illustrates how:

• A good response to clozapine may be achieved in a patient whose illness has shown only a limited response to first-line antipsychotic treatment (see Chapter 6).
• Cardiac side effects can limit the use of clozapine (see Chapter 7).
• High-dose and combination antipsychotic treatment generally have limited clinical benefit, although are widely used in clinical practice. It is recommended that these strategies are not routinely used and, if they are tried, each use is treated as an individual therapeutic trial (see Chapter 9).

Case 11: A case illustrating therapeutic strategies in a patient who has shown limited response to clozapine

Thomas R. E. Barnes

A 36-year-old female patient with a diagnosis of treatment-resistant schizophrenia reported a 2-month history of increasing auditory hallucinations, voices that were critical and distressing. There was no evidence of significant depressive or anxiety symptoms or other psychotic symptoms. She had been prescribed clozapine for the past 5 years and assured her psychiatrist that she adhered well to this medication. She was a non-smoker. Her serum clozapine level was checked and was within the suggested therapeutic range. Increasing the dose of clozapine did not improve her symptoms but led to constipation and sedation, side effects that resolved with a return to the previous dose. The voices continued and a decision was made to augment the clozapine with amisulpride. Six months later, there had been no change in the auditory hallucinations but the patient reported that her periods had stopped shortly after starting amisulpride. The serum prolactin level was found to be markedly elevated and this was attributed to the addition of amisulpride. Given the lack of evident benefit with this augmentation strategy, the amisulpride was discontinued. Distraction techniques were employed to try and reduce the impact of the patient's voices in terms of distress and disability. Soon after, the auditory hallucinations reduced in severity, which may have partly reflected the psychological intervention but also a concurrent reduction in her cannabis use. She denied drinking alcohol excessively or using any other street drugs currently or at any time recently, but cannabis use was judged to have contributed to the deterioration in her illness in the past year.

CHAPTER 13

Learning points

This case illustrates:

- The approach to establishing an adequate trial of clozapine (see Chapter 6).
- The use of clozapine augmentation with a second antipsychotic (see Chapter 12).
- The importance of addressing comorbid factors (see Chapter 2).
- The potential value of psychological approaches (see Chapter 11).

Case 12: A case illustrating the potential of cognitive behavioural therapy for psychosis to target resistant psychosis

Majella Byrne, Suzanne Jolley, and Emmanuelle Peters

Jane is a 41-year-old white British woman, who was diagnosed with schizophrenia at age 19 years. She lives with her husband and her two children, aged 9 and 7 years. Her husband is 25 years her senior. Jane is a shy and timid person. She describes her husband as overbearing and controlling and she is afraid to challenge him or go against his wishes. She was an only child and described her upbringing as conventional. She described her parents as religious, harsh, critical, overprotective, and domineering. She reported that they encouraged her not to trust others. Jane experiences commanding voices, one male and one female, who make negative comments about her and tell her to harm herself by cutting. She has complied with the voices in the past, cutting her arms and legs with a razor blade. Jane is well engaged with mental health services and is compliant with antipsychotic medication, but the voices have remained. She has noticed that, at times when she has forgotten to take her medication, the voices become louder and more distracting and she also experiences derealization, which she finds distressing. Jane experiences the voices as powerful, critical, and threatening. She believes that she has no control over the voices, she feels powerless and worthless, and she does not believe she would be able to stand up to them for fear of the consequences. She worries that if she does not comply with the voices, they will be displeased, become louder and more critical and could harm her. Her relationship with the voices is similar to the relationship she has with others, including her parents and husband, where she takes a subordinate position. Jane has a deep-rooted belief that she is a bad person, deserving punishment, and that others are more powerful than her. Jane's mood is generally low and she has distressing intrusive thoughts about jumping in front of a moving train. She avoids walking too close to the edge of the platform and prefers to have someone with her when travelling by train. Jane expects others to think badly of her, to be critical and judgemental. Jane hears the voices daily.

When in the supermarket she frequently hears them over the tannoy. At home she hears them coming from the radio in her kitchen and she hears them when in the bathroom. Jane's belief in the power of the voices maintains her harmful compliance, which reinforces her beliefs that she deserves to be punished, that she is powerless and unable to cope. Jane was referred for cognitive behavioural therapy for psychosis (CBTp) by her psychiatrist. Her goals for therapy include understanding her voices and gaining support to try to change how she responds to voices. She is motivated to begin therapy at this point because she is becoming increasingly worried about the impact of her difficulties on her children, particularly on her son, who is struggling with separation anxiety and finds it difficult to be apart from his mother, even for brief periods. The sessions have helped her to understand the vicious cycle of thoughts, behaviours, and symptoms, and how these reinforce each other (Fig. 13.1). They have also helped her to develop alternative responses (exits from the vicious cycle; Fig. 13.1).

Learning points

- Jane's case illustrates ongoing, distressing psychotic experiences despite some benefit from antipsychotic treatment (see Chapter 3).
- Her life experiences have contributed to beliefs that she is powerless to stand up for herself, which means she feels compelled to act on hallucinatory experiences telling her to harm herself; this illustrates how beliefs can influence the impact of psychosis (see Chapter 11).
- She also believes that she is a bad person and deserves punishment. These beliefs are echoed in the content of the voices she hears, leading to low mood (see Chapter 11).
- CBTp will aim to target her behavioural response to the voices and the underlying beliefs that maintain these, to help her cope and function better (see Fig. 13.1 and Chapter 11).

Case 13: A case of antipsychotic non-adherence illustrating the potential of cognitive behavioural therapy for psychosis to target cognitive and behavioural factors maintaining psychosis

Majella Byrne, Suzanne Jolley, and Emmanuelle Peters

Eduardo is a 38-year-old single Brazilian man who has been living in the UK for 8 years. Eduardo has a diagnosis of paranoid schizophrenia and he had his first episode 10 years previously. He grew up in an urban area in a family of limited means. He described his father and two sisters as 'bullying' throughout his childhood, while he reported his mother to be a source of comfort and protection. He reported that he was bullied at school by people he had initially thought were friends.

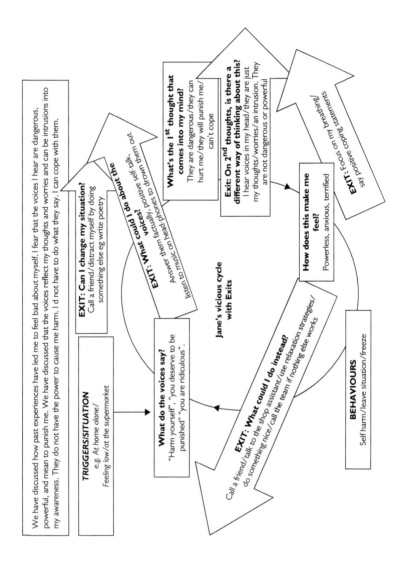

We have discussed how past experiences have led me to feel bad about myself. I fear that the voices I hear are dangerous, powerful, and mean to punish me. We have discussed that the voices reflect my thoughts and worries and can be intrusions into my awareness. They do not have the power to cause me harm. I d not have to do what they say. I can cope with them.

TRIGGERS/SITUATION
e.g. At home alone/
Feeling low/at the supermarket

EXIT: Can I change my situation?
Call a friend/distract myself by doing
something else eg write poetry

EXIT: What could I do about the voices?
Answer them factually, positive self-talk,
listen to music on head-phones to drown them out

What's the 1st thought that comes into my mind?
They are dangerous/they can hurt me/they will punish me/
can't cope

Exit: On 2nd thoughts, is there a different way of thinking about this?
I hear voices in my head/they are just my thoughts/worries/an intrusion. They are not dangerous or powerful

How does this make me feel?
Powerless, anxious, terrified

EXIT: Focus on my breathing/
say positive coping statements

Jane's vicious cycle with Exits

What do the voices say?
"Harm yourself", "you deserve to be punished" "you are ridiculous".

EXIT: What could I do instead?
Call a friend/talk to the shop assistant/ use relaxation strategies/
do something nice/ call the team if nothing else works

BEHAVIOURS
Self harm/leave situation/freeze

Fig. 13.1 Jane's vicious cycle with exits.

He said that he has always found it difficult to read other peoples' intentions. He is a religious man and is a member of the Jehovah Witness church. Eduardo has had two admissions to hospital in the UK, the last of which was 4 years ago. He refuses to take antipsychotic medication as he has reported that it has the effect of dulling his emotions. He is engaged with services and is happy to contact them for support when he is struggling to cope. Within the past 2 years Eduardo has experienced a number of difficult life events, including being beaten up at his gym in an unprovoked attack and discovering that his girlfriend had been cheating on him. These experiences further cemented his beliefs that people cannot be trusted, that there are dangerous psychopaths all around, and that he has to be very careful to protect himself from them. He believes that psychopaths will manipulate his feelings and lead him to feel humiliated, ashamed, and rejected. Eduardo works as a cleaner and does not have much interaction with colleagues during the day. He lives alone in a bedsit and has few friends. He speaks to his mother approximately once a week by telephone. He has no other family contacts. When Eduardo is out of the house he feels anxious in anticipation of meeting psychopaths who could hurt him. Therefore, to maximize his safety, he scans the faces of the people he sees around him, he listens carefully to the words people use in conversation, and he observes their body language to aid him in identifying psychopaths. While he still attends church, he has become less sociable in interactions with others there, being careful not to give too much away about himself for fear of being hurt. Eduardo is angry with his neighbour, who he believes is trying to annoy him by playing loud music and making other noises in the evening. Eduardo displays a strong jumping-to-conclusions cognitive bias, a personalizing bias, and a concrete thinking style. While alone, he often ruminates on past experiences of bullying and his vulnerability to being targeted by psychopaths. This has the effect of lowering his mood and motivation, and leads to him feeling bad about himself. It also increases his hypervigilance to signs that people could be psychopaths. Eduardo was referred to therapy by his psychiatrist. His goals for therapy are to improve his personal relationships, to be more assertive in relationships, and to improve his lifestyle and personal wellbeing. During sessions with his therapist, Eduardo identified the vicious cycle of thoughts, feelings, and behaviours that was maintaining his symptoms and the triggers to the cycle (Fig. 13.2). He went on to develop and try out alternative thoughts and responses (exits in Fig. 13.2).

Learning points

- Side effects of antipsychotic treatment, including subjective effects (as is the case here), may outweigh their benefits for some patients (see Chapters 3 and 7).
- Eduardo's case illustrates how early life experiences, such as being bullied as a child, can lead to ways of thinking, such as 'there are dangerous psychopaths all around', that can underlie and reinforce delusions (see Chapter 11).

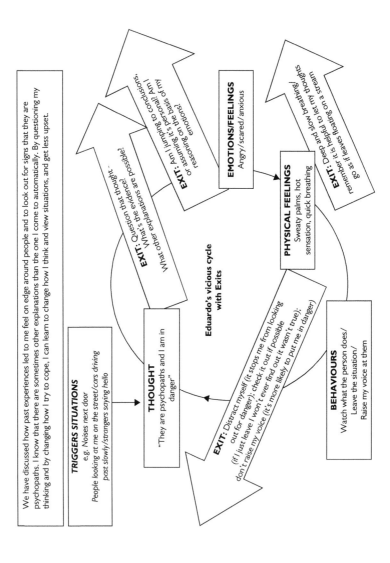

We have discussed how past experiences led to me feel on edge around people and to look out for signs that they are psychopaths. I know that there are sometimes other explanations than the one I come to automatically. By questioning my thinking and by changing how I try to cope, I can learn to change how I think and view situations, and get less upset.

TRIGGERS SITUATIONS
e.g. Noises next door
People looking at me on the street/cars driving past slowly/strangers saying hello

THOUGHT
"They are psychopaths and I am in danger"

EXIT: Question that thought – What's the evidence? What other explanations are possible!

EXIT: Am I jumping to conclusions. Am I assuming it's personal? Am I 'assuming on the basis of my reasoning emotions?

EMOTIONS/FEELINGS
Angry/scared/anxious

PHYSICAL FEELINGS
Sweaty palms, hot sensation, quick breathing

EXIT: Deep and slow breathing/ remember it is helpful to let my thoughts go as if leaves floating on a stream

Eduardo's vicious cycle with Exits

EXIT: Distract myself (it stops me from looking out for danger); check it out if possible (if I just leave I won't ever find out if possible don't raise my voice (it's more likely to put me in danger)

BEHAVIOURS
Watch what the person does/ Leave the situation/ Raise my voice at them

Fig. 13.2 Eduardo's vicious cycle with exits.

- This case also illustrates safety behaviours, such as actively looking for signs that others may be psychopaths and being socially reserved, that may serve to reinforce delusions (see Chapter 11).

- With his cognitive behavioural therapy for psychosis therapist he will target safety behaviours and consider more helpful responses and alternatives to his beliefs that psychopaths are all around (Fig. 13.2).

Case 14: A case of late-onset treatment resistance

Robert McCutcheon, Christoph U. Correll, Oliver Howes, and John Kane

Mr Smith initially responded to long-acting injectable antipsychotic treatment well, and as a result of improvements in his functioning he was able to move out of the family home into an independent accommodation, and was subsequently discharged from mental health services to his general practitioner. He was re-referred to the community psychiatric team 5 years later. The referral letter noted that his family members were concerned owing to increasing social withdrawal, poor functioning, and increased suspiciousness. A home visit was undertaken, and the decision was made to increase the dose of his flupentixol decanoate i.m. On review 2 months later, extrapyramidal side effects were apparent, and there had still not been significant improvement to Mr Smith's mental state. As a result, a change to oral olanzapine was undertaken under the supervision of a home treatment team, who administered treatment directly to him, ensuring adherence. Six weeks of treatment at 20 mg per day had minimal impact, and a diagnosis of late-onset treatment resistance was made. Following discussion with Mr Smith and his family, a trial of clozapine was undertaken. The home treatment team administered clozapine and this was titrated to 500 mg per day, which corresponded to a plasma level of 0.4 µg/L. Mr Smith described himself as feeling 'calmer' on clozapine and was keen to continue treatment. He was able to continue clozapine treatment without further home treatment team input, maintaining plasma levels above 0.35 µg/L. His family and clinical team noted a marked improvement in his mental state, with a reduction in suspiciousness, and a return to previous levels of social interaction and functioning.

Learning points

- Medication response can diminish over time, leading to the development of late or secondary treatment resistance (see Chapter 2).

- Clozapine should be considered even in patients who have shown difficulties maintaining adherence in the past. Adjustments may be needed (e.g. mobile phone prompts or in-person supervision), although in some cases an improvement in mental state may lead to improved ability to adhere to treatment (see Chapter 6).

Case 15: A case illustrating clozapine-eligible treatment-resistant schizophrenia

Gary Remington, Ofer Agid, Hiroyoshi Takeuchi, Jimmy Lee, and Araba Chintoh

The patient is a 48-year-old gentleman whose psychiatric history dates back to early adulthood. At that time, he was attending university and he reported increasing paranoia, referential ideas, grandiosity, and perceptual disturbances (both visual and auditory). During that same period, he drank in excess frequently and used street drugs, predominantly marijuana. He dropped out of university that year and since has been unable to work or return to school.

There is no medical history of note beyond the substance abuse, and no known family psychiatric history. Since his first psychotic break, he has required four hospitalizations over the years, although none in the past decade. He has been treated with numerous psychotropics and his current daily medications include olanzapine 20 mg/day, haloperidol 4 mg/day, clonazepam 1 mg/day, and citalopram 30 mg/day. He attends no programmes, socializes little, and lives in supportive housing.

Notably, he did undergo a trial of clozapine during the second decade of his illness. The dose was gradually increased to 125 mg daily over the first 2 weeks but he discontinued the trial because of subjective sedation. Notes related to that trial do not report any added benefits related to clozapine, with the caveat that the trial was inadequate in terms of both dose and duration.

Currently, he attends monthly appointments but otherwise remains largely isolated, staying in his room. He presents as somewhat dishevelled, although he regularly attends his appointments and is cooperative during assessments. He demonstrates poor insight regarding his symptoms and his thought form is both loose and tangential on occasion. When he has enough funds, he drinks alcohol to excess, and this occurs 3–4 times monthly. He can become confrontational at times, which is linked to his paranoia and referential ideas. He does not become assaultive but is threatening. He hears voices almost continuously and on occasion experiences visual hallucinations.

He remains on the aforementioned medication regime and reports no side effects. He has had multiple antipsychotic trials over the years, including long-acting injectable antipsychotics earlier in the course of his illness, a point when non-adherence was a significant issue. This is not seen to be an issue any longer, but continued efforts to switch antipsychotics are tempered by documented lack of response to numerous non-clozapine agents to this point as well as his reluctance to change his present medications. Repeated efforts have been made to have him undertake another trial of clozapine as, at this point, he remains clozapine-eligible in the face of an inadequate trial.

Learning points

• Comorbid harmful substance use may contribute to treatment resistance by worsening symptoms and reducing treatment adherence (see Chapter 2). Treating substance use can be effective where the patient will engage in treatment.

• Both the dose and duration of clozapine treatment in this case is inadequate, and this case cannot thus be considered to have a clozapine-resistant (ultra-medication treatment-resistant) illness (see Chapters 2 and 12).

• Side effects such as sedation are often prominent early in the initiation of clozapine, and can lead to early discontinuation if not proactively managed (see Chapter 7).

• Proactive management of side effects is recommended to support a patient to remain on clozapine for an adequate trial (see Chapter 7).

Case 16: A case of clozapine (ultra-medication)-resistant schizophrenia

Gary Remington, Ofer Agid, Hiroyoshi Takeuchi, Jimmy Lee, and Araba Chintoh

The patient is a 30-year-old single Caucasian male with a psychiatric history dating back to mid-adolescence. Changes were noted at that time, including decreased performance at school, trouble concentrating, religious preoccupation, and assaultive behaviour. Substance abuse was not identified as an issue, and there was no noted family psychiatric history. He dropped out of school within 1–2 years, at which point he lived at home and did not work.

An additional assault led to his referral for psychiatric care, and he was hospitalized involuntarily for assessment. At that time, symptoms of psychosis were identified, including paranoia, referential ideas, grandiosity, and perceptual disturbances (e.g. hearing voices).

Treatment was initiated with an oral antipsychotic and he improved to the point where he could be discharged. However, shortly after leaving hospital he became non-adherent and was rehospitalized. Over the next several years, adequate trials of other oral antipsychotics were initiated but, once again, non-adherence was an issue outside of hospital. Long-acting injectable antipsychotics were also used to address the non-adherence, but symptoms persisted even in the face of several adequate long-acting injectable antipsychotic drug trials, allowing for the diagnosis of clozapine-eligible schizophrenia (or treatment-resistant schizophrenia).

At this point clozapine was raised as a treatment option, although he had now been ill for several years. At the point that clozapine was suggested, he had entered the forensic system and was once again hospitalized following further legal charges that led to him being assessed as NCR (not criminally responsible).

Clozapine doses were increased over the next months, but psychotic symptoms remained. Therapeutic drug monitoring indicated that plasma clozapine levels were well within the recommended therapeutic thresholds, and the dose was increased up to 900 mg daily in an effort to achieve response. However, he remained quite symptomatic.

In addition to high-dose clozapine, efforts focused on clozapine augmentation were undertaken. This included various antipsychotics being added to clozapine, including haloperidol, sulpiride, and aripiprazole, mood stabilizers (valproate), and bilateral electroconvulsive therapy with little clear benefit.

He has now been in hospital for several years and remains NCR within the forensic system. While adherence is closely monitored in hospital, as evidenced by clozapine levels that are consistently within the recommended therapeutic thresholds, he remains quite psychotic. Currently, he meets criteria for clozapine-resistant schizophrenia, and none of the augmentation strategies to date has proven effective. In fact, the question has been raised as to whether clozapine warrants continuation. He has now developed metabolic side effects related to clozapine treatment, including weight gain and type 2 diabetes requiring treatment. However, clozapine did produce at least partial response, reflected in notable clinical worsening when he discontinued it at one point.

Learning points

- Significant psychotic symptoms persist despite clozapine doses at the top of the licensed dose range and plasma clozapine levels well within recommended therapeutic plasma levels, indicating clozapine resistance (see Chapter 12).
- The evidence for clozapine augmentation strategies is limited and, where they are used, they should be considered as an individual therapeutic trial, with careful evaluation of clinical response and side effects (see Chapter 12).
- Response to clozapine may be inadequate, as shown by marked, persistent symptoms and impairment, but nevertheless there may be some benefit from clozapine, and a worsening on its discontinuation, as is the case here. The limited benefit from clozapine should be carefully evaluated against the risk of side effects.

Case 17: A case of clozapine (ultra-medication)-resistant schizophrenia with onset in adolescence

Robert McCutcheon, Christoph U. Correll, Oliver Howes, and John Kane

Ms Brown was seen by child and adolescent mental health services at age 17 owing to declining academic performance, and bizarre behaviour noted by her school teachers and family. She was accompanied by her father, who revealed that both her mother and maternal aunt had diagnoses of schizophrenia. Clinical assessment determined that she had been experiencing auditory hallucinations for the past 2 months, and that she had developed persecutory delusional beliefs regarding several of her friends. A diagnosis of schizophreniform disorder was felt to be most likely, and treatment with risperidone 0.5 mg/day was commenced. This was gradually increased to 6 mg/day over the next 3 months, but no improvement in her positive psychotic symptoms was observed, and both negative and cognitive symptoms appeared to be worsening, despite her father administering treatment, ensuring adherence. Inpatient admission was arranged and a trial of olanzapine was undertaken for 6 weeks, with doses increased from 10 to 20 mg/day. No improvement was seen, and Ms Brown requested to change medication owing to significant weight gain. Over the following 2 years, Ms Brown underwent trials of amisulpride and aripiprazole, neither of which significantly improved her mental state. The potential risk and benefits of clozapine treatment were discussed with Ms Brown, and the decision was made to commence treatment in conjunction with metformin given her history of antipsychotic-induced weight gain. Clozapine was initiated in the community, with the dose gradually increasing from 12.5 mg to 450 mg over the course of 6 weeks. Plasma level testing revealed levels consistently greater than 0.4 µg/L. No objective or subjective improvement was noted in symptoms and so the dose was increased to 600 mg, with valproic acid added for seizure prophylaxis. Ms Brown continued to show minimal improvement in her symptoms despite clozapine treatment for over 6 months, with plasma levels consistently >0.4 µg/L, suggesting a clozapine (ultra-medication)-resistant form of illness, which prompted discussions about a trial of electroconvulsive therapy.

Learning points

- A proportion of patients, about 60%, will not respond to clozapine treatment (see Chapter 12). Careful assessment of mental state is recommended both before and after clozapine treatment to allow an informed decision regarding the risk–benefit balance of continuing treatment in cases of minimal response (see Chapter 2).
- Where clozapine (ultra-medication) resistance has been established, adjunctive and alternative treatments may be warranted, although the evidence base is limited (see Chapter 12).

CHAPTER 14

Novel treatments and future directions

Seiya Miyamoto and Nobumi Miyake

KEY POINTS

- There are considerable medical needs not met by current antipsychotic treatment, particularly for patients with negative symptoms and cognitive impairments, and for treatment-resistant schizophrenia.

- A growing body of research has identified new molecular mechanisms, neural systems, and novel pharmacological targets for treating schizophrenia beyond just dopamine D2 antagonism.

- Drugs in development include compounds targeting novel dopaminergic approaches, including preferential D1 antagonism for treatment resistance, and partial agonists for negative symptoms.

- Glutamatergic and cholinergic approaches have been positive in some studies, but results of drugs in large clinical trials have been disappointing so far.

- Cannabinoid, anti-inflammatory, neurosteroid, and a number of other approaches have shown promising initial results.

- There is also evidence to support a number of non-pharmacological strategies, including computer-based avatar therapy, cognitive remediation, and neurostimulatory approaches.

Introduction

The advent of new-generation antipsychotic drugs (APDs) has broadened the options for the pharmacological treatment of schizophrenia (Miyake et al., 2012). Moreover, a growing body of research has identified new molecular mechanisms and novel pharmacological targets beyond dopamine D2 antagonism (Miyamoto et al., 2013; 2012; Fleischhacker and Miyamoto, 2016). However, there are still unmet medical needs in the current antipsychotic treatment, particularly for patients with negative symptoms and cognitive impairments, and for patients with treatment-resistant schizophrenia (TRS). In the following sections, we consider compounds under development grouped by their main putative brain target.

New dopaminergic approaches

All currently approved APDs have dopamine D2 antagonistic activity (Miyamoto et al., 2014). Numerous dopaminergic agents that are not primarily D2 antagonists have also been developed, including D1 antagonists (e.g. SCH39166 and ADX-1006/NNC 01-0687), D1/D2 agonists (e.g. dihydrexidine and lisdexamfetamine), D3 antagonists (e.g. ABT-925), and D4 antagonists (e.g. fananserin, sonepiprazole, and L-745,870) (Miyamoto et al., 2012). However, the results of clinical trials of these compounds to date have been inconclusive and none has yet been licensed for schizophrenia.

Dopamine D2/D3 partial agonists such as aripiprazole, brexpiprazole, and cariprazine (all currently licensed) may stabilize dopamine function. RP5063 is another under development which has partial agonist activity and has shown promise in a phase 2 trial (Cantillon et al., 2017).

Another dopaminergic drug under development is Lu AF35700. This has a novel pharmacological profile with predominant D1 versus D2 antagonistic activity (Fellner, 2017). It is also an antagonist of the serotonin (5-HT)2A and 5-HT6 receptors. A phase 3 trial of Lu AF35700 is under way in patients with TRS.

Glutamatergic approaches

N-methyl-D-aspartate receptor (NMDA-R) hypofunction has been proposed to contribute to the pathophysiology of schizophrenia (Javitt and Zukin, 1991; Coyle, 1996; Krystal et al., 1994). Moreover, NMDA-R hypofunction may result in compensatory excessive glutamatergic neurotransmission at non-NMDA receptors (Kantrowitz and Javitt, 2012). Compounds that enhance NMDA-R activity, including glycine site modulators (e.g. glycine, D-serine, D-cycloserine, and D-alanine) and glycine reuptake inhibitors (e.g. sarcosine, bitopertin, and AMG 747), have been evaluated for their potential in treating schizophrenia (Javitt and Zukin, 1991; Coyle, 1996; Krystal et al., 1994; Miyamoto et al., 2012; Umbricht et al., 2014; Dunayevich et al., 2017). Other glutamatergic agents include metabotropic glutamate receptor agonists (e.g. pomaglumetad methionil), metabotropic glutamate receptor modulators (e.g. ADX47273 and JNJ-40411813/ADX71149), ampakines (e.g. CX516 and farampator), and α-amino-3-hydroxy-5-methyl-4-isoxazolepropionic acid (AMPA) receptor potentiators (e.g. PF-04958242) (Miyamoto et al., 2012). Unfortunately, the results of clinical studies of these agents thus far have not been promising (Stauffer et al., 2013; Bugarski-Kirola et al., 2017).

Cannabinoids

Acute cannabis intoxication and chronic cannabis use can produce psychotic symptoms, and long-term cannabis use can increase the risk of psychotic disorders

(Gage et al., 2016). Growing evidence suggests that the endocannabinoid system, including cannabinoid-1 receptors and anandamide, an endocannabinoid transmitter, may be related to the regulation of mood and cognition (Di Marzo and Petrosino, 2007). As such, pharmacological modulation of this system has been suggested to represent a potential new therapeutic target in schizophrenia (Rohleder et al., 2016; Zamberletti et al., 2012).

Cannabidiol (CBD), the largest phytochemical component of cannabis, does not have psychotomimetic effects or induce dependence following chronic use (Ligresti et al., 2016). A number of preclinical studies have demonstrated that CBD has anti-inflammatory, neuroprotective, antidepressant, and antipsychotic properties (Campos et al., 2017; Rohleder et al., 2016; Seeman, 2016). In a phase 2 double-blind randomized controlled trial (RCT), CBD showed antipsychotic properties equivalent to amisulpride in patients with acutely exacerbated schizophrenia (Leweke et al., 2012). CBD was well tolerated and demonstrated a superior adverse effect profile compared with that of amisulpride. It is notable that CBD increased serum anandamide levels, and these were correlated with clinical improvement. However, in another double-blind RCT, CBD did not show improvement in selective attention in patients with schizophrenia (Hallak et al., 2010). Whilst promising, further studies are needed with larger sample sizes and longer durations of treatment to determine whether CBD has beneficial effects on psychotic and/or cognitive symptoms of schizophrenia.

Cholinergic drugs

Nicotinic acetylcholine receptors (nAChRs) have a key role in the regulation of attention, memory, and sensory gating (Wallace et al., 2011). Among nAChRs, the α_7 nAChR subtype is the drug target of greatest interest for treating schizophrenia. Selective α_7 nAChR agonists such as 3-2,4-dimethoxybenzylidene anabaseine (DMXB-A), RG3487 (MEM3454), EVP-6124 (encenicline), tropisetron, TC-5619, ABT-126, and AQW-051 have been developed as potential candidates for adjunctive treatments of cognitive impairment and negative symptoms in schizophrenia (Hashimoto, 2015; Kantrowitz, 2017). Whilst demonstrating potential benefits of encenicline on cognition and negative symptoms in a phase 2b study (Keefe et al., 2015), phase 3 trials have not confirmed such efficacy (Keshavan et al., 2017). Similarly, although adjunctive TC-5619 improved executive function and negative symptoms in a phase 2a study (Lieberman et al., 2013), the results of a phase 2 trial of TC-5619 did not support such efficacy in schizophrenia (Walling et al., 2016).

Another nAChR with a significant role in cognition is the $\alpha_4 \beta_2$ subtype. Agonists at this receptor such as AZD3480 (TC-1734), varenicline, SIB-1553A, and RJR2403 have been tested as adjunctive agents to APDs for cognitive impairment associated with schizophrenia (CIAS) (Gray and Roth, 2007; Arneric et al., 2007). However, the results have so far proven inconclusive (Smith et al., 2016; Velligan et al., 2012).

Neurosteroids

Neuroactive steroids, or neurosteroids, including pregnenolone, pregnenolone sulfate, allopregnanolone, dehydroepiandrosterone (DHEA), and DHEA sulfate, have been suggested to have neuroprotective and neurotrophic properties and have a variety of functions related to stress response, mood regulation, and cognitive performance (Maninger et al., 2009; Ritsner, 2011). Among neurosteroids, pregnenolone and DHEA may be promising therapeutic candidates in schizophrenia (Marx et al., 2011).

Initial findings of clinical trials of pregnenolone demonstrated significant efficacy on negative, positive, and cognitive symptoms in patients with schizophrenia or schizoaffective disorder (Marx et al., 2009; Ritsner et al., 2010). However, subsequent studies yielded inconsistent results (Kashani et al., 2017; Kardashev et al., 2018; Marx et al., 2014; Ritsner et al., 2014; Kreinin et al., 2017). Thus far, there are also conflicting data regarding the potential clinical benefits of adjunctive DHEA on the treatment of schizophrenia (Strous et al., 2003; 2007; Nachshoni et al., 2005; Ritsner et al., 2006; 2010). Further long-term large studies of neurosteroids are warranted with broader dose ranges.

Novel anti-inflammatory and related strategies

Accumulating evidence suggests that inflammation, immune system dysfunction, and oxidative stress may be implicated in the pathogenesis of schizophrenia (Feigenson et al., 2014; Keshavan et al., 2017; Miller and Buckley, 2016). Moreover, novel lines of evidence from genetics have shown that alterations in the complement system are related to the illness (Sekar et al., 2016), and this system can regulate microglial activity and synaptic pruning (Stephan et al., 2012). Overactivated microglia may lead to accelerated pruning of synapses and loss of cortical grey matter (Howes and McCutcheon, 2017).

Various anti-inflammatory strategies such as cyclooxygenase-1/2 inhibitors (e.g. celecoxib and aspirin), minocycline, and monoclonal antibodies (e.g. tocilizumab) have been investigated in clinical trials in schizophrenia (Nitta et al., 2013; Na et al., 2014; Miller et al., 2016). However, in a meta-analysis of adjunctive use of non-steroidal anti-inflammatory drugs (NSAIDs) for schizophrenia, NSAIDs were not superior to placebo in Positive And Negative Syndrome Scale (PANSS) total or negative symptom scores (Nitta et al., 2013).

Minocycline has anti-inflammatory, antioxidant, and neuroprotective properties, probably through nitric oxide synthase inhibition, inhibition of microglial activation, and antiapoptotic properties (Plane et al., 2010). Two recent meta-analyses of RCTs showed beneficial effects of adjunctive minocycline on general psychopathology and negative symptoms in patients with schizophrenia (Solmi et al., 2017; Xiang et al., 2017). It is suggested that anti-inflammatory strategies might be most effective early in disease progression (Kenk et al., 2015; Keshavan et al., 2017).

Adjunctive monoclonal antibody immunotherapy in schizophrenia may have advantages over other anti-inflammatory approaches. For example, monoclonal antibodies are less likely to have off-target (non-immune) effects and they are more specific because they act by neutralizing inflammatory cytokines or by binding cytokine receptors (Miller and Buckley, 2016). Research on monoclonal antibody immunotherapy could clarify a possible role of inflammation in the pathophysiology of schizophrenia. On the other hand, potential serious adverse effects (e.g. infections and malignancy) and the high cost of such therapy may limit use in clinical practice (Miller and Buckley, 2016).

It has been proposed that deficits in glutathione, an endogenous antioxidant, are involved in the pathophysiology of schizophrenia and they may impair myelination processes and white matter maturation (Monin et al., 2015; Keshavan et al., 2017). Acetylcysteine (also referred to as N-acetylcysteine (NAC)), a glutathione precursor, has potent antioxidant, proneurogenesis, and anti-inflammatory properties and appears to be safe and tolerable (Deepmala et al., 2015). Two RCTs showed the efficacy of adjunctive NAC on clinical symptoms in patients with chronic schizophrenia (Berk et al., 2008; Farokhnia et al., 2013). Further studies are warranted to confirm the findings.

Other pharmacological approaches

Serotonin (5-HT) receptors have been proposed as a target for the efficacy of APDs and the development of new agents (Stone and Pilowsky, 2007). Serotonergic approaches for the treatment of schizophrenia include 5-HT1A agonists, 5-HT reuptake inhibitors, 5-HT2A antagonists and inverse agonists, 5-HT2C antagonists and agonists, 5-HT3 antagonists, 5-HT6 antagonists, and 5-HT7 antagonists (Keshavan et al., 2017). Various agents, either as monotherapy or in combination with D2 antagonism and/or 5-HT2A antagonism, are in different stages of development. For example, pimavanserin, an inverse agonist at the 5HT2A receptor, was approved for the treatment of psychosis associated with Parkinson's disease (Howland, 2016). Adjunctive pimavanserin had shown promise in a phase 2 trial in patients with chronic schizophrenia (Meltzer et al., 2012), and phase 3 studies are under way. MIN-101 is a 5-HT2A and sigma-2 receptor antagonist (Fellner, 2017) and, in a phase 2b trial, it showed efficacy for negative symptoms of schizophrenia (Davidson et al., 2017).

Gamma-aminobutyric acid (GABA) is the major inhibitory neurotransmitter of the central nervous system (CNS), and GABA-mediated hypoactivity has been of interest in the pathophysiological mechanism of schizophrenia (Wassef et al., 2003). Efforts to develop GABAergic agents such as selective GABA type A (GABA$_A$) receptor agonists (e.g. MK-0777), GABA type B (GABA$_B$) receptor antagonists, and allosteric modulators at GABA$_A$ receptor subtypes (alpha 1, 2, 3, and 5) are under way (Keshavan et al., 2017).

Phosphodiesterase 10A (PDE10A) is a dual specificity enzyme that hydrolyses both cAMP and cGMP (Kehler and Kilburn, 2009). PDE10A inhibitors, including papaverine, TP-10, MP-10, TAK-063, JNJ-42314415, RO5545965, THPP-1, and PDM-042, demonstrated antipsychotic-like effects in animal models of schizophrenia (Kehler and Kilburn, 2009; Grauer et al., 2009). However, the results of clinical trials of PDE10A inhibitors thus far have not been promising (Dunlop and Brandon, 2015).

Elevated brain levels of kynurenic acid (KYNA), a metabolite of tryptophan, have been linked to CIAS (Wu et al., 2014). KYNA is reported to inhibit NMDA-Rs and α_7 nAChRs (Kozak et al., 2014). Kynurenine aminotransferase (KAT) II, the enzyme responsible for brain KYNA neosynthesis, has been proposed as a potential new target for the treatment of CIAS (Kozak et al., 2014; Wu et al., 2014). Studies of KAT II inhibitors (e.g. PF-04859989, (S)-4-(ethylsulfonyl) benzoylalanine, and BFF-816) are under way.

Non-pharmacological approaches

AVATAR therapy (audiovisual-assisted therapy aid for refractory auditory hallucinations) has recently been developed as a novel computer-assisted psychological intervention for the management of medication-resistant auditory hallucinations (Leff et al., 2013). In the therapy, each patient can create the AVATAR as an external computer-generated entity and interact it. The therapist can control the AVATAR and change its character from being abusive to becoming friendly and helpful, so that the patient gradually achieves control over their AVATAR and raises their self-esteem (Leff et al., 2014). In a recent RCT, AVATAR therapy for 12 weeks demonstrated promising effects on refractory auditory hallucinations (Craig et al., 2018), and a further trial is now under way.

Several epidemiological studies have linked schizophrenia to coeliac disease, which is an immune-mediated enteropathy induced by the ingestion of gluten-containing grains (Kalaydjian et al., 2006). Up to one-quarter of patients with schizophrenia have been reported to possess antibodies to gliadin (Jin et al., 2012; Cascella et al., 2011). An open-label pilot study demonstrated that a gluten-free diet resulted in improvement in schizophrenic symptoms and extrapyramidal side effects in patients with antibodies to antibodies to gliadin or antitissue transglutaminase (Jackson et al., 2012). Further research is necessary to examine the effect of a gluten-free diet on symptoms in antibody-positive patients with schizophrenia.

Electroconvulsive therapy (ECT) has shown promise as an effective and safe strategy for the short-term treatment of patients with clozapine-resistant TRS (Lally et al., 2016). It has generally been given alongside clozapine in patients with clozapine-resistant schizophrenia in open-label studies, with evidence of clinical benefits. However, further research is needed to confirm its long-term effects and the need for maintenance treatments (Miyamoto et al., 2015). Two meta-analyses of RCTs of repetitive transcranial magnetic stimulation (rTMS) suggest that it may have short-term efficacy for medication-resistant verbal auditory hallucinations in schizophrenia (Slotema et al., 2014; 2012). However, it remains unknown whether rTMS as monotherapy is more effective than rTMS as an adjunctive to clozapine (Miyamoto et al., 2015). Transcranial direct current stimulation (tDCS) is another non-invasive brain stimulation technique. Compared with ECT and rTMS, tDCS is more convenient and less expensive (Miyamoto et al., 2015). To date, three RCTs of tDCS have been conducted to evaluate its effects on verbal auditory hallucinations (Brunelin et al., 2012; Frohlich et al., 2016; Smith et al., 2015). However, the sample sizes of these trials were small and the results were inconsistent (Li et al., 2016). A further review of other non-pharmacological approaches such as neuromodulation and psychosocial interventions can be found in recent articles (Miyamoto et al., 2015; Nieuwdorp et al., 2015; Lynch et al., 2010; Wykes et al., 2011).

Cognitive remediation (CR) is another behavioural intervention aiming to improve cognitive function (Cella et al., 2017). The meta-analyses of RCTs suggest that CR has beneficial effects on global cognition and function in patients with schizophrenia with small-to-moderate effect sizes (Wykes et al., 2011), and this effect may be associated with activation of the frontal and parietal lobe (Wei et al., 2016). CR may also have a small-to-moderate effect on negative symptoms of schizophrenia (Cella et al., 2017).

New approaches to treatment

At present, a number of different compounds with novel targets are in different stages of drug development (Table 14.1). However, none has thus far definitively been proven effective for schizophrenia, particularly for negative symptoms and CIAS (Correll et al., 2017).

Patients with schizophrenia show considerable variations in their response to treatments and there is no reliable method to predict such differences (Joyce et al., 2017). This individual heterogeneity may be affected by diverse factors such as age, gender, race, genetics, pathophysiology, comorbidities, and environmental interactions (Keshavan et al., 2017; Miyamoto et al., 2012; Tandon et al., 2010). Our current, symptom-based diagnostic strategy may result in aetiological and pathophysiological heterogeneity (Keshavan et al., 2017; Clementz et al., 2016). Dysfunction in specific systems or circuits may occur in subsets of patients with schizophrenia, which could influence the likelihood of response to specific treatments (Insel, 2012). Identification of the molecular mechanisms that have an effect on individual responsiveness to treatment is warranted to establish effective personalized care (Rogers and Goldsmith, 2009).

The National Institute of Mental Health in the USA has developed the Research Domain Criteria (RDoC) project to incorporate genetic and neurobiological information into a system-based dimension rather than categorical diagnostic system (Insel, 2014; Insel et al., 2010). The RDoC approach may help to deconstruct schizophrenia into translational units of analyses (Keshavan et al., 2017), and eventually facilitate understanding of the aetiology, pathogenesis, and heterogeneity of the illness, hopefully linking understanding at the level of molecule, circuit,

Table 14.1 New drug target and compounds for the treatment of schizophrenia

Mechanism of action	Compound	Main result and/or status
Dopaminergic agents		
D1 antagonist	SCH39166	Discontinuation of development
	ADX-10061/NNC 01-0687	Discontinuation of development
	Lu AF35700	In phase 3
D1/D2 agonist	dihydrexidine	Further studies required
	lisdexamfetamine	Discontinuation of development
D2/D3 partial agonist	RP5063	Phase 3 study in preparation
D3 antagonist	ABT-925	Discontinuation of development
D4 antagonist	fananserin	Discontinuation of development
	sonepiprazole	Discontinuation of development
	L-745,870	Negative results
Glutamatergic agents		
Glycine site modulator	glycine	No further development
	D-serine	No further development
	D-cycloserine	No further development
	D-alanine	No further development
Glycine reuptake inhibitor	sarcosine	No further development
	bitopertin	Discontinuation of development after phase 3
	AMG 747	Discontinuation of development
Metabotropic glutamate receptor agonist	pomaglumetad methionil	Discontinuation of development after phase 3
Metabotropic glutamate receptor modulator	ADX47273	In early development
	JNJ-40411813/ADX71149	In early development

continued >

Table 14.1 New drug target and compounds for the treatment of schizophrenia *(continued)*

Ampakine	CX516	Discontinuation of development
	farampator	In early development
AMPA receptor potentiator	PF-04958242	Phase 2 study terminated
Cannabinoids		
	cannabidiol	Results of a phase 2 study awaited
Cholinergic agents		
Selective α_7 nAChR agonist	DMXB-A	Discontinuation of development
	RG3487 (MEM3454)	Discontinuation of development
	EVP-6124 (encenicline)	Discontinuation of development after phase 3
	tropisetron	Results of a large RCT awaited
	TC-5619	Mixed results thus far
	ABT-126	Discontinuation of development
	AQW-051	Results of an RCT awaited
$\alpha_4 \beta_2$ nAChR agonist	AZD3480 (TC-1734)	Negative results in a phase 2 study
	varenicline	Negative effects on cognition
	SIB-1553A	In early development
	RJR2403	In early development
Neurosteroids		
	pregnenolone	Mixed results thus far
	dehydroepiandrosterone	Mixed results thus far

continued >

NOVEL TREATMENTS AND FUTURE DIRECTIONS • 193

Anti-inflammatory agents		
Antioxidant and neuroprotective	minocyclin	Further studies required
	acetylcysteine	Further studies required
Cyclooxygenase-1/2 inhibitor	celecoxib	Mixed results thus far
	aspirin	Mixed results thus far
Monoclonal antibody	tocilizumab	Further studies required
Miscellaneous agents		
5-HT2A inverse agonist	pimavanserin	In phase 3
5-HT2A and sigma-2 antagonist	MIN-101	In phase 3
GABA$_A$ receptor agonist	MK-0777	Little benefit for cognitive impairment
Phosphodiesterase 10A inhibitor	papaverine	Discontinuation of development
	TP-10	In early development
	MP-10	In early development
	TAK-063	Results of a phase 2 study awaited
	JNJ-42314415	In early development
	RO5545965	Results of a phase 1 study awaited
	THPP-1	In early development
	PDM-042	In early development
Kynurenine aminotransferase II inhibitor	PF-04859989	In early development
	(S)-4-(ethylsulfonyl) benzoylalanine	In early development
	BFF-816	In early development
RCT, Randomized controlled trials.		

behaviour, and symptom (Kim et al., 2017). Such approaches should help the development of hypothesis-driven targeted drug treatments for schizophrenia.

There is also a great need for the development of translational biomarkers such as imaging and physiological measures based on novel pathophysiological models to show target engagement (Keshavan et al., 2017; Insel, 2012; Millan et al., 2015). In future clinical trials, novel treatments are likely to be focused on specific patient subgroups based on profiling and the identification of endophenotypes using reliable biomarkers. Clinical implementation of such practices could permit stratification of patient populations and have a strong impact on improving treatment efficacy and reducing adverse effects, moving towards precision medicine (Arranz and de Leon, 2007; Insel, 2012).

Conclusions

The limitations of current antipsychotic treatments discussed in previous chapters highlights that there is an urgent need for the development of new agents with superior efficacy and fewer side effects. This is most marked for treatment resistance, where there is only one licensed drug, clozapine. A number of compounds with novel mechanisms of action have been explored and evaluated in recent years. So far, several new dopaminergic (e.g. RP5063 and Lu AF35700), serotonergic (e.g. pimavanserin and MIN-101), and anti-inflammatory (e.g. minocycline and NAC) compounds in development show promise as therapeutic candidates in schizophrenia and are undergoing clinical trials. A number of adjunctive non-pharmacological strategies under evaluation, such as neuromodulation (e.g. ECT and rTMS) and psychosocial interventions (e.g. AVATAR therapy and CR), also show promise. It is important to consider patient selection strategies in future clinical trials to improve the evaluation of new treatments. Effective biomarkers would not only improve the drug development process but also facilitate personalized medicine by better identifying the appropriate patient subgroups that might respond to specific treatments. Furthermore, a more complete understanding of the pathophysiology of schizophrenia informed by translational research is essential to discover novel targets with potentially disease-modifying treatments and to identify the ideal time and duration of intervention.

REFERENCES

Arneric, S. P., Holladay, M., Williams, M. (2007). Neuronal nicotinic receptors: a perspective on two decades of drug discovery research. *Biochem Pharmacol,* 74, 1092–101.

Arranz, M. J., de Leon, J. (2007). Pharmacogenetics and pharmacogenomics of schizophrenia: a review of last decade of research. *Mol Psychiatry,* 12, 707–47.

Berk, M., Copolov, D., Dean, O., et al. (2008). N-acetyl cysteine as a glutathione precursor for schizophrenia—a double-blind, randomized, placebo-controlled trial. *Biol Psychiatry,* 64, 361–8.

Brunelin, J., Mondino, M., Gassab, L., et al. (2012). Examining transcranial direct-current stimulation (tDCS) as a treatment for hallucinations in schizophrenia. *Am J Psychiatry*, 169, 719–24.

Bugarski-Kirola, D., Blaettler, T., Arango, C., et al. (2017). Bitopertin in negative symptoms of schizophrenia—results from the phase III FlashLyte and DayLyte studies. *Biol Psychiatry*, 82, 8–16.

Campos, A. C., Fogaca, M. V., Scarante, F. F., et al. (2017). Plastic and neuroprotective mechanisms involved in the therapeutic effects of cannabidiol in psychiatric disorders. *Front Pharmacol*, 8, 269.

Cantillon, M., Prakash, A., Alexander, A., Ings, R., Sweitzer, D., Bhat, L. (2017). Dopamine serotonin stabilizer RP5063: a randomized, double-blind, placebo-controlled multicenter trial of safety and efficacy in exacerbation of schizophrenia or schizoaffective disorder. *Schizophr Res*, 189, 126–33.

Cascella, N. G., Kryszak, D., Bhatti, B., et al. (2011). Prevalence of celiac disease and gluten sensitivity in the United States clinical antipsychotic trials of intervention effectiveness study population. *Schizophr Bull*, 37, 94–100.

Cella, M., Preti, A., Edwards, C., Dow, T., Wykes, T. (2017). Cognitive remediation for negative symptoms of schizophrenia: a network meta-analysis. *Clin Psychol Rev*, 52, 43–51.

Clementz, B. A., Sweeney, J. A., Hamm, J. P., et al. (2016). Identification of distinct psychosis biotypes using brain-based biomarkers. *Am J Psychiatry*, 173, 373–84.

Correll, C. U., Rubio, J. M., Inczedy-Farkas, G., Birnbaum, M. L., Kane, J. M., Leucht, S. (2017). Efficacy of 42 pharmacologic cotreatment strategies added to antipsychotic monotherapy in schizophrenia: systematic overview and quality appraisal of the meta-analytic evidence. *JAMA Psychiatry*, 74, 675–84.

Coyle, J. T. (1996). The glutamatergic dysfunction hypothesis for schizophrenia. *Harv Rev Psychiatry*, 3, 241–53.

Craig, T. K., Rus-Calafell, M., Ward, T., et al. (2018). AVATAR therapy for auditory verbal hallucinations in people with psychosis: a single-blind, randomised controlled trial. *Lancet Psychiatry*, 5, 31–40.

Davidson, M., Saoud, J., Staner, C., et al. (2017). Efficacy and safety of MIN-101: a 12-week randomized, double-blind, placebo-controlled trial of a new drug in development for the treatment of negative symptoms in schizophrenia. *Am J Psychiatry*, 174, 1195–202.

Deepmala, Slattery, J., Kumar, N., et al. (2015). Clinical trials of N-acetylcysteine in psychiatry and neurology: a systematic review. *Neurosci Biobehav Rev*, 55, 294–321.

Di Marzo, V., Petrosino, S. (2007). Endocannabinoids and the regulation of their levels in health and disease. *Curr Opin Lipidol*, 18, 129–40.

Dunayevich, E., Buchanan, R. W., Chen, C. Y., et al. (2017). Efficacy and safety of the glycine transporter type-1 inhibitor AMG 747 for the treatment of negative symptoms associated with schizophrenia. *Schizophr Res*, 182, 90–7.

Dunlop, J., Brandon, N. J. (2015). Schizophrenia drug discovery and development in an evolving era: are new drug targets fulfilling expectations? *J Psychopharmacol*, 29, 230–8.

Farokhnia, M., Azarkolah, A., Adinehfar, F., et al. (2013). N-acetylcysteine as an adjunct to risperidone for treatment of negative symptoms in patients with chronic schizophrenia: a randomized, double-blind, placebo-controlled study. *Clin Neuropharmacol*, 36, 185–92.

Feigenson, K. A., Kusnecov, A. W., Silverstein, S. M. (2014). Inflammation and the two-hit hypothesis of schizophrenia. *Neurosci Biobehav Rev*, 38, 72–93.

Fellner, C. (2017). New schizophrenia treatments address unmet clinical needs. *P T*, 42, 130–4.

Fleischhacker, W. W., Miyamoto, S. (2016). Pharmacological treatment of schizophrenia: current issues and future perspectives. *Clin Neuropsychopharmacol Therapeut*, 7, 1–8.

Frohlich, F., Burrello, T. N., Mellin, J. M., et al. (2016). Exploratory study of once-daily transcranial direct current stimulation (tDCS) as a treatment for auditory hallucinations in schizophrenia. *Eur Psychiatry*, 33, 54–60.

Gage, S. H., Hickman, M., Zammit, S. (2016). Association between cannabis and psychosis: epidemiologic evidence. *Biol Psychiatry*, 79, 549–56.

Grauer, S. M., Pulito, V. L., Navarra, R. L., et al. (2009). Phosphodiesterase 10A inhibitor activity in preclinical models of the positive, cognitive, and negative symptoms of schizophrenia. *J Pharmacol Exp Ther*, 331, 574–90.

Gray, J. A., Roth, B. L. (2007). Molecular targets for treating cognitive dysfunction in schizophrenia. *Schizophr Bull*, 33, 1100–19.

Hallak, J. E., Machado-De-Sousa, J. P., Crippa, J. A., et al. (2010). Performance of schizophrenic patients in the Stroop Color Word Test and electrodermal responsiveness after acute administration of cannabidiol (CBD). *Rev Bras Psiquiatr*, 32, 56–61.

Hashimoto, K. (2015). Targeting of alpha7 nicotinic acetylcholine receptors in the treatment of schizophrenia and the use of auditory sensory gating as a translational biomarker. *Curr Pharm Des*, 21, 3797–806.

Howes, O. D., McCutcheon, R. (2017). Inflammation and the neural diathesis-stress hypothesis of schizophrenia: a reconceptualization. *Transl Psychiatry*, 7, e1024.

Howland, R. H. (2016). Pimavanserin: an inverse agonist antipsychotic drug. *J Psychosoc Nurs Ment Health Serv*, 54, 21–4.

Insel, T., Cuthbert, B., Garvey, M., et al. (2010). Research domain criteria (RDoC): toward a new classification framework for research on mental disorders. *Am J Psychiatry*, 167, 748–51.

Insel, T. R. (2012). Next-generation treatments for mental disorders. *Sci Transl Med*, 4, 155ps19.

Insel, T. R. (2014). The NIMH Research Domain Criteria (RDoC) Project: precision medicine for psychiatry. *Am J Psychiatry*, 171, 395–7.

Jackson, J., Eaton, W., Cascella, N., et al. (2012). A gluten-free diet in people with schizophrenia and anti-tissue transglutaminase or anti-gliadin antibodies. *Schizophr Res*, 140, 262–3.

Javitt, D. C., Zukin, S. R. (1991). Recent advances in the phencyclidine model of schizophrenia. *Am J Psychiatry*, 148, 1301–8.

Jin, S. Z., Wu, N., Xu, Q., et al. (2012). A study of circulating gliadin antibodies in schizophrenia among a Chinese population. *Schizophr Bull*, 38, 514–18.

Joyce, D. W., Kehagia, A. A., Tracy, D. K., Proctor, J., Shergill, S. S. (2017). Realising stratified psychiatry using multidimensional signatures and trajectories. *J Transl Med*, 15, 15.

Kalaydjian, A. E., Eaton, W., Cascella, N., Fasano, A. (2006). The gluten connection: the association between schizophrenia and celiac disease. *Acta Psychiatr Scand*, 113, 82–90.

Kantrowitz, J., Javitt, D. C. (2012). Glutamatergic transmission in schizophrenia: from basic research to clinical practice. *Curr Opin Psychiatry*, 25, 96–102.

Kantrowitz, J. T. (2017). Managing negative symptoms of schizophrenia: how far have we come? *CNS Drugs*, 31, 373–88.

Kardashev, A., Ratner, Y., Ritsner, M. S. (2018). Add-on pregnenolone with L-theanine to antipsychotic therapy relieves negative and anxiety symptoms of schizophrenia: an 8-week, randomized, double-blind, placebo-controlled trial. *Clin Schizophr Relat Psychoses*, 12, 31–41.

Kashani, L., Shams, N., Moazen-Zadeh, E., et al. (2017). Pregnenolone as an adjunct to risperidone for treatment of women with schizophrenia: a randomized double-blind placebo-controlled clinical trial. *J Psychiatr Res*, 94, 70–7.

Keefe, R. S., Meltzer, H. A., Dgetluck, N., et al. (2015). Randomized, double-blind, placebo-controlled study of encenicline, an alpha7 nicotinic acetylcholine receptor agonist, as a treatment for cognitive impairment in schizophrenia. *Neuropsychopharmacology*, 40, 3053–60.

Kehler, J., Kilburn, J. P. (2009). Patented PDE10A inhibitors: novel compounds since 2007. *Expert Opin Ther Pat*, 19, 1715–25.

Kenk, M., Selvanathan, T., Rao, N., et al. (2015). Imaging neuroinflammation in gray and white matter in schizophrenia: an in-vivo PET study with [18F]-FEPPA. *Schizophr Bull*, 41, 85–93.

Keshavan, M. S., Lawler, A. N., Nasrallah, H. A., Tandon, R. (2017). New drug developments in psychosis: challenges, opportunities and strategies. *Prog Neurobiol*, 152, 3–20.

Kim, Y. K., Choi, J., Park, S. C. (2017). A novel bio-psychosocial-behavioral treatment model in schizophrenia. *Int J Mol Sci*, 18, pii: E734.

Kozak, R., Campbell, B. M., Strick, C. A., et al. (2014). Reduction of brain kynurenic acid improves cognitive function. *J Neurosci*, 34, 10592–602.

Kreinin, A., Bawakny, N., Ritsner, M. S. (2017). Adjunctive pregnenolone ameliorates the cognitive deficits in recent-onset schizophrenia: an 8-week, randomized, double-blind, placebo-controlled trial. *Clin Schizophr Relat Psychoses*, 10, 201–10.

Krystal, J. H., Karper, L. P., Seibyl, J. P., et al. (1994). Subanesthetic effects of the noncompetitive NMDA antagonist, ketamine, in humans. Psychotomimetic, perceptual, cognitive, and neuroendocrine responses. *Arch Gen Psychiatry*, 51, 199–214.

Lally, J., Tully, J., Robertson, D., Stubbs, B., Gaughran, F., Maccabe, J. H. (2016). Augmentation of clozapine with electroconvulsive therapy in treatment resistant schizophrenia: a systematic review and meta-analysis. *Schizophr Res*, 171, 215–24.

Leff, J., Williams, G., Huckvale, M. A., Arbuthnot, M., Leff, A. P. (2013). Computer-assisted therapy for medication-resistant auditory hallucinations: proof-of-concept study. *Br J Psychiatry*, 202, 428–33.

Leff, J., Williams, G., Huckvale, M., Arbuthnot, M., Leff, A. P. (2014). Avatar therapy for persecutory auditory hallucinations: what is it and how does it work? *Psychosis*, 6, 166–76.

Leweke, F. M., Piomelli, D., Pahlisch, F., et al. (2012). Cannabidiol enhances anandamide signaling and alleviates psychotic symptoms of schizophrenia. *Transl Psychiatry*, 2, e94.

Li, H., Wang, Y., Jiang, J., Li, W., Li, C. (2016). Effects of transcranial direct current stimulation (tDCS) for auditory hallucinations: a systematic review. *Shanghai Arch Psychiatry*, 28, 301–8.

Lieberman, J. A., Dunbar, G., Segreti, A. C., et al. (2013). A randomized exploratory trial of an alpha-7 nicotinic receptor agonist (TC-5619) for cognitive enhancement in schizophrenia. *Neuropsychopharmacology*, 38, 968–75.

Ligresti, A., De Petrocellis, L., Di Marzo, V. (2016). From phytocannabinoids to cannabinoid receptors and endocannabinoids: pleiotropic physiological and pathological roles through complex pharmacology. *Physiol Rev*, 96, 1593–659.

Lynch, D., Laws, K. R., Mckenna, P. J. (2010). Cognitive behavioural therapy for major psychiatric disorder: does it really work? A meta-analytical review of well-controlled trials. *Psychol Med*, 40, 9–24.

Maninger, N., Wolkowitz, O. M., Reus, V. I., Epel, E. S., Mellon, S. H. (2009). Neurobiological and neuropsychiatric effects of dehydroepiandrosterone (DHEA) and DHEA sulfate (DHEAS). *Front Neuroendocrinol*, 30, 65–91.

Marx, C. E., Keefe, R. S., Buchanan, R. W., et al. (2009). Proof-of-concept trial with the neurosteroid pregnenolone targeting cognitive and negative symptoms in schizophrenia. *Neuropsychopharmacology*, 34, 1885–903.

Marx, C. E., Bradford, D. W., Hamer, R. M., et al. (2011). Pregnenolone as a novel therapeutic candidate in schizophrenia: emerging preclinical and clinical evidence. *Neuroscience*, 191, 78–90.

Marx, C. E., Lee, J., Subramaniam, M., et al. (2014). Proof-of-concept randomized controlled trial of pregnenolone in schizophrenia. *Psychopharmacology (Berl)*, 231, 3647–62.

Meltzer, H. Y., Elkis, H., Vanover, K., et al. (2012). Pimavanserin, a selective serotonin (5-HT)2A-inverse agonist, enhances the efficacy and safety of risperidone, 2 mg/day, but does not enhance efficacy of haloperidol, 2 mg/day: comparison with reference dose risperidone, 6 mg/day. *Schizophr Res*, 141, 144–52.

Millan, M. J., Goodwin, G. M., Meyer-Lindenberg, A., Ove Ogren, S. (2015). Learning from the past and looking to the future: emerging perspectives for improving the treatment of psychiatric disorders. *Eur Neuropsychopharmacol*, 25, 599–656.

Miller, B. J., Buckley, P. F. (2016). The case for adjunctive monoclonal antibody immunotherapy in schizophrenia. *Psychiatr Clin North Am*, 39, 187–98.

Miller, B. J., Dias, J. K., Lemos, H. P., Buckley, P. F. (2016). An open-label, pilot trial of adjunctive tocilizumab in schizophrenia. *J Clin Psychiatry*, 77, 275–6.

Miyake, N., Miyamoto, S., Jarskog, L. F. (2012). New serotonin/dopamine antagonists for the treatment of schizophrenia: are we making real progress? *Clin Schizophr Relat Psychoses*, 6, 122–33.

Miyamoto, S., Miyake, N., Jarskog, L. F., Fleischhacker, W. W., Lieberman, J. A. (2012). Pharmacological treatment of schizophrenia: a critical review of the pharmacology and clinical effects of current and future therapeutic agents. *Mol Psychiatry*, 17, 1206–27.

Miyamoto, S., Jarskog, L. F., Fleischhacker, W. W. (2013). Alternative pharmacologic targets for the treatment of schizophrenia: results from phase I and II trials. *Curr Opin Psychiatry*, 26, 158–65.

Miyamoto, S., Merrill, D. B., Jarskog, L. F., Fleishhacker, W. W., Marder, S. R., Lieberman, J. A. (2014). Antipsychotic drugs. In: Tasman, A., Kay, J., Lieberman, J. A., First, M. B., Riba, M. B. (eds) *Psychiatry*, 4th edn. Chichester: John Wiley & Sons, Ltd.

Miyamoto, S., Jarskog, L. F., Fleischhacker, W. W. (2015). Schizophrenia: when clozapine fails. *Curr Opin Psychiatry*, 28, 243–8.

Monin, A., Baumann, P. S., Griffa, A., et al. (2015). Glutathione deficit impairs myelin maturation: relevance for white matter integrity in schizophrenia patients. *Mol Psychiatry*, 20, 827–38.

Na, K. S., Jung, H. Y., Kim, Y. K. (2014). The role of pro-inflammatory cytokines in the neuroinflammation and neurogenesis of schizophrenia. *Prog Neuropsychopharmacol Biol Psychiatry*, 48, 277–86.

Nachshoni, T., Ebert, T., Abramovitch, Y., et al. (2005). Improvement of extrapyramidal symptoms following dehydroepiandrosterone (DHEA) administration in antipsychotic treated schizophrenia patients: a randomized, double-blind placebo controlled trial. *Schizophr Res*, 79, 251–6.

Nieuwdorp, W., Koops, S., Somers, M., Sommer, I. E. (2015). Transcranial magnetic stimulation, transcranial direct current stimulation and electroconvulsive therapy for medication-resistant psychosis of schizophrenia. *Curr Opin Psychiatry*, 28, 222–8.

Nitta, M., Kishimoto, T., Muller, N., et al. (2013). Adjunctive use of nonsteroidal anti-inflammatory drugs for schizophrenia: a meta-analytic investigation of randomized controlled trials. *Schizophr Bull*, 39, 1230–41.

Plane, J. M., Shen, Y., Pleasure, D. E., Deng, W. (2010). Prospects for minocycline neuroprotection. *Arch Neurol*, 67, 1442–8.

Ritsner, M. S. (2011). The clinical and therapeutic potentials of dehydroepiandrosterone and pregnenolone in schizophrenia. *Neuroscience*, 191, 91–100.

Ritsner, M. S., Gibel, A., Ratner, Y., Tsinovoy, G., Strous, R. D. (2006). Improvement of sustained attention and visual and movement skills, but not clinical symptoms, after dehydroepiandrosterone augmentation in schizophrenia: a randomized, double-blind, placebo-controlled, crossover trial. *J Clin Psychopharmacol*, 26, 495–9.

Ritsner, M. S., Gibel, A., Shleifer, T., et al. (2010). Pregnenolone and dehydroepiandrosterone as an adjunctive treatment in schizophrenia and schizoaffective disorder: an 8-week, double-blind, randomized, controlled, 2-center, parallel-group trial. *J Clin Psychiatry*, 71, 1351–62.

Ritsner, M. S., Bawakny, H., Kreinin, A. (2014). Pregnenolone treatment reduces severity of negative symptoms in recent-onset schizophrenia: an 8-week, double-blind, randomized add-on two-center trial. *Psychiatry Clin Neurosci*, 68, 432–40.

Rogers, D. P., Goldsmith, C. A. (2009). Treatment of schizophrenia in the 21st century: beyond the neurotransmitter hypothesis. *Expert Rev Neurother*, 9, 47–54.

Rohleder, C., Muller, J. K., Lange, B., Leweke, F. M. (2016). Cannabidiol as a potential new type of an antipsychotic. A critical review of the evidence. *Front Pharmacol*, 7, 422.

Seeman, P. (2016). Cannabidiol is a partial agonist at dopamine D2 high receptors, predicting its antipsychotic clinical dose. *Transl Psychiatry*, 6, e920.

Sekar, A., Bialas, A. R., De Rivera, H., et al. (2016). Schizophrenia risk from complex variation of complement component 4. *Nature*, 530, 177–83.

Slotema, C. W., Aleman, A., Daskalakis, Z. J., Sommer, I. E. (2012). Meta-analysis of repetitive transcranial magnetic stimulation in the treatment of auditory verbal hallucinations: update and effects after one month. *Schizophr Res*, 142, 40–5.

Slotema, C. W., Blom, J. D., Van Lutterveld, R., Hoek, H. W., Sommer, I. E. (2014). Review of the efficacy of transcranial magnetic stimulation for auditory verbal hallucinations. *Biol Psychiatry*, 76, 101–10.

Smith, R. C., Boules, S., Mattiuz, S., et al. (2015). Effects of transcranial direct current stimulation (tDCS) on cognition, symptoms, and smoking in schizophrenia: a randomized controlled study. *Schizophr Res*, 168, 260–6.

Smith, R. C., Amiaz, R., Si, T. M., et al. (2016). Varenicline effects on smoking, cognition, and psychiatric symptoms in schizophrenia: a double-blind randomized trial. *PLoS One*, 11, e0143490.

Solmi, M., Veronese, N., Thapa, N., et al. (2017). Systematic review and meta-analysis of the efficacy and safety of minocycline in schizophrenia. *CNS Spectr*, 22, 415–26.

Stauffer, V. L., Millen, B. A., Andersen, S., et al. (2013). Pomaglumetad methionil: no significant difference as an adjunctive treatment for patients with prominent negative symptoms of schizophrenia compared to placebo. *Schizophr Res*, 150, 434–41.

Stephan, A. H., Barres, B. A., Stevens, B. (2012). The complement system: an unexpected role in synaptic pruning during development and disease. *Annu Rev Neurosci*, 35, 369–89.

Stone, J. M., Pilowsky, L. S. (2007). Novel targets for drugs in schizophrenia. *CNS Neurol Disord Drug Targets*, 6, 265–72.

Strous, R. D., Maayan, R., Lapidus, R., et al. (2003). Dehydroepiandrosterone augmentation in the management of negative, depressive, and anxiety symptoms in schizophrenia. *Arch Gen Psychiatry*, 60, 133–41.

Strous, R. D., Stryjer, R., Maayan, R., et al. (2007). Analysis of clinical symptomatology, extrapyramidal symptoms and neurocognitive dysfunction following dehydroepiandrosterone (DHEA) administration in olanzapine treated schizophrenia patients: a randomized, double-blind placebo controlled trial. *Psychoneuroendocrinology*, 32, 96–105.

Tandon, R., Nasrallah, H. A., Keshavan, M. S. (2010). Schizophrenia, 'just the facts' 5. Treatment and prevention. Past, present, and future. *Schizophr Res*, 122, 1–23.

Umbricht, D., Alberati, D., Martin-Facklam, M., et al. (2014). Effect of bitopertin, a glycine reuptake inhibitor, on negative symptoms of schizophrenia: a randomized, double-blind, proof-of-concept study. *JAMA Psychiatry*, 71, 637–46.

Velligan, D., Brenner, R., Sicuro, F., et al. (2012). Assessment of the effects of AZD3480 on cognitive function in patients with schizophrenia. *Schizophr Res*, 134, 59–64.

Wallace, T. L., Ballard, T. M., Pouzet, B., Riedel, W. J., Wettstein, J. G. (2011). Drug targets for cognitive enhancement in neuropsychiatric disorders. *Pharmacol Biochem Behav*, 99, 130–45.

Walling, D., Marder, S. R., Kane, J., et al. (2016). Phase 2 trial of an alpha-7 nicotinic receptor agonist (TC-5619) in negative and cognitive symptoms of schizophrenia. *Schizophr Bull*, 42, 335–43.

Wassef, A., Baker, J., Kochan, L. D. (2003). GABA and schizophrenia: a review of basic science and clinical studies. *J Clin Psychopharmacol*, 23, 601–40.

Wei, Y. Y., Wang, J. J., Yan, C., et al. (2016). Correlation between brain activation changes and cognitive improvement following cognitive remediation therapy in schizophrenia: an activation likelihood estimation meta-analysis. *Chin Med J (Engl)*, 129, 578–85.

Wu, H. Q., Okuyama, M., Kajii, Y., Pocivavsek, A., Bruno, J. P., Schwarcz, R. (2014). Targeting kynurenine aminotransferase II in psychiatric diseases: promising effects of an orally active enzyme inhibitor. *Schizophr Bull*, 40 (Suppl. 2), S152–8.

Wykes, T., Huddy, V., Cellard, C., McGurk, S. R., Czobor, P. (2011). A meta-analysis of cognitive remediation for schizophrenia: methodology and effect sizes. *Am J Psychiatry*, 168, 472–85.

Xiang, Y. Q., Zheng, W., Wang, S. B., et al. (2017). Adjunctive minocycline for schizophrenia: a meta-analysis of randomized controlled trials. *Eur Neuropsychopharmacol*, 27, 8–18.

Zamberletti, E., Rubino, T., Parolaro, D. (2012). The endocannabinoid system and schizophrenia: integration of evidence. *Curr Pharm Des*, 18, 4980–90.

Index

Note: *b* denotes box, *f* figure and *t* is table